'This is a wonderful palmistry book, especially for astrologers schooled in the Hindu/Vedic system known as Jyotish. There is a wealth of knowledge here for anyone who wishes to delve deeper into the subject than has ever been possible. The text is easy to understand, clear and precise, comprehensive and well-researched. While there are many modern palmistry books, as well as the older ones by Cheiro, on the market, this text exceeds those by leaps and bounds, incorporating rich, detailed ancient Vedic writings. Andrew Mason, who studied Jyotish and palmistry in Sri Lanka with several teachers, appears to have written something of a masterpiece!'

– *James Braha, Vedic Astrologer*

'There are many systems for reading the palm, including Indian, Chinese, Greek and others, yet the situation of *prakāśagrahas* (sun and moon), *târâ-graha* (planets), *tamograha* (nodes) and *nakshatras* (stars) provide the means by which palmists seek to divine the future. Other practitioners of palmistry solely use meditative power, performing *Karña Pishācinī Siddhī* at sunrise before consulting the palm. *Vedic Palmistry: Hastā Rekha Shāstra* succeeds in giving a detailed account of these ancient practices. With easy-to-follow text and clear illustrations, rekhas (lines), grahas (planets) and rashis (zodiacal signs) are all skilfully brought into the light of understanding.'

– *Professor Hari Shankara Sharma, PhD, Āyurveda – Post Graduation Studies and Research (IPGT&R) Gujarat Āyurveda University (Ret).*

by the same author

Jyotish
The Art of Vedic Astrology
Foreword by James Braha
ISBN 978 1 84819 210 2
eISBN 978 0 85701 160 2

Rasa Shastra
The Hidden Art of Medical Alchemy
ISBN 978 1 84819 107 5
eISBN 978 0 85701 088 9

of related interest

Vital Healing
Energy, Mind and Spirit in Traditional Medicines of India, Tibet and the Middle East - Middle Asia
Marc S. Micozzi, MD, PhD with Donald McCown and Mones Abu-Asab, PhD (Unani), Hakima Amri, PhD (Unani), Kevin Ergil, MA, MS, LAc (Tibet), Howard Hall, PsyD, PhD (Sufi), Hari Sharma, MD (Maharishi Ayurveda), Kenneth G. Zysk, DPhil, PhD (Ayurveda & Siddha)
ISBN 978 1 84819 045 0 (hardback)
ISBN 978 1 84819 156 3 (paperback)
eISBN 978 0 85701 025 4

Ayurvedic Medicine
The Principles of Traditional Practice
Sebastian Pole
ISBN 978 1 84819 113 6
eISBN 978 0 85701 091 9

Ayurvedic Healing
Contemporary Maharishi Ayurveda Medicine and Science, Second Edition
Hari Sharma, MD and Christopher Clark, MD
ISBN 978 1 84819 069 6
eISBN 978 0 85701 063 6

Alchemy of Pushing Hands
Oleg Tcherne
ISBN 978 1 84819 022 1
eISBN 978 0 85701 003 2

Vedic Palmistry

Hastā Rekha Shāstra

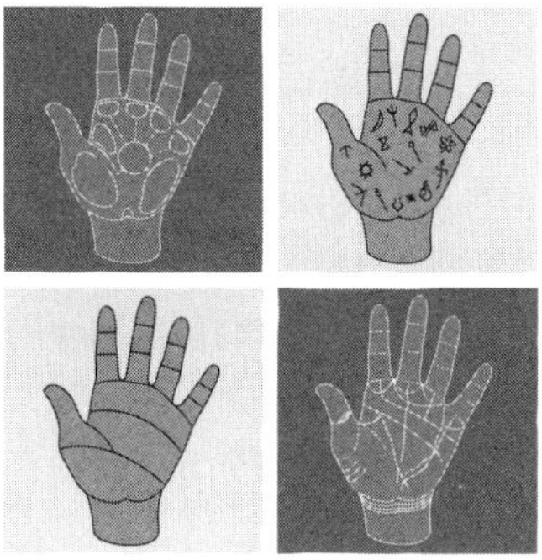

ANDREW MASON

SINGING
DRAGON
LONDON AND PHILADELPHIA

First published in 2017
by Singing Dragon
an imprint of Jessica Kingsley Publishers
73 Collier Street
London N1 9BE, UK
and
400 Market Street, Suite 400
Philadelphia, PA 19106, USA

www.singingdragon.com

Library of Congress Cataloging in Publication Data
A CIP catalog record for this book is available from the Library of Congress

British Library Cataloguing in Publication Data
A CIP catalogue record for this book is available from the British Library

ISBN 978 1 84819 350 5
eISBN 978 0 85701 309 5

Printed and bound in Great Britain

FSC www.fsc.org
MIX
Paper from responsible sources
FSC® C013056

Dedicated to my wife Atsuko
and daughter Himiko

ACKNOWLEDGEMENTS

The author would like to extend his appreciation to the following people, without whom this book could not have been written:

My sincere thanks go to Philip Weeks, Dr Mauroof Athique, Meulin Athique, Udaya Dandunnage, Ātreya Smith, Edith Hathaway and Oliver Sabetian.

With special thanks to James Braha, Professor Hari Shankara Sharma, Victoria Peters, Andrew Kirk, Dagmar Wujastyk, Ilona Kędzia, Dr V. N. Joshi, Shamala Joshi, Utkoor Yajna Narayana Purohit and Jessica Kingsley.

CONTENTS

VEDIC PALMISTRY

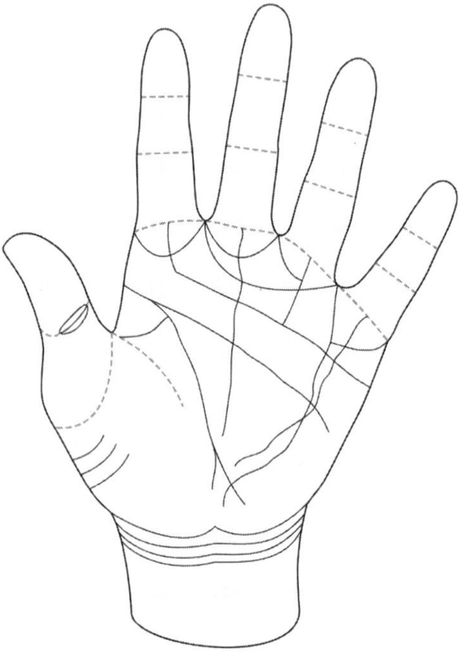

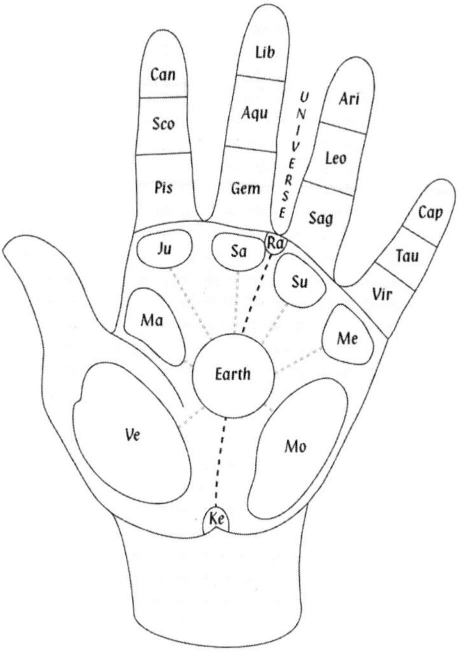
Can
Sco
Pis
Lib
Aqu
Gem
UNIVERSE
Ari
Leo
Sag
Cap
Tau
Vir
Ju
Sa
Ra
Su
Ma
Me
Earth
Ve
Mo
Ke

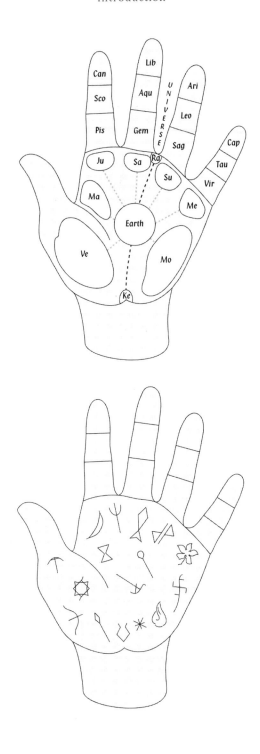

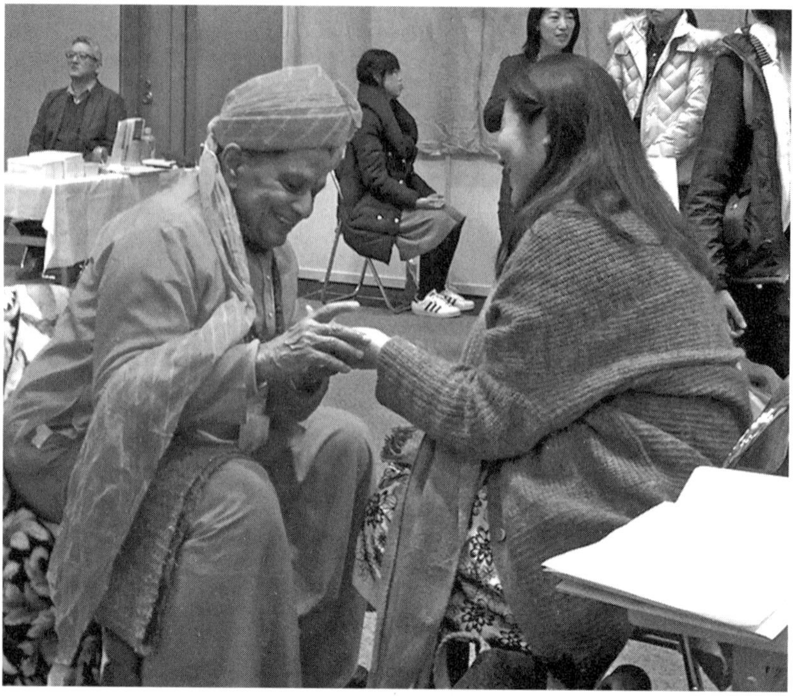

Traditional Indian Astro-palmist examining a client's palm.

> A line originating from the root of the youngest finger indicates a life of a hundred years. If a line passes from the tip of the thumb to that of the forefinger it indicates shortness of life. If a line originates from the foot of the thumb and is long it indicates the possession of sons and if short indicates the possession of women.
>
> *Garuda Puṛāna*

Mention anything astrological in Śrī Laṇkā or India and fully expect to have your listener wave his or her palm under your nose, inquiring as to their prospects for wealth, health, longevity, spouse and progeny. Here astrology and palmistry are quite simply inseparable[1] as any Jyotishi (astrologer) worth his salt is expected to have a good working knowledge of both. To the ancients, the hand, or more specifically its lines, detailed the will of the nine planets in their roles of karmic emissaries.

Unlike astrology, palmistry requires little understanding of planetary motion, transits or the construction of horoscopes. As we carry our hands about our person, our destiny is readily accessible, should we happen to cross the path of one adept in palmistry. This is not to say the aforementioned knowledge should be absent, as many times those skilled in palm analysis corroborate any statements with a cursory glance at their client's horoscope, or vice versa. Considered in unison, each complements one another very nicely.

Akin to precepts of Vedic Astrology (Jyotish) and traditional Indian Medicine (Āyurveda), among others, palmistry can appear quite simplistic to an onlooker, its core principles easily grasped within a few hours of study. However, successful application of these sciences can be the work of multiple lifetimes.

SIGNS UPON THE BODY

It does not seem possible to credit any one nation or people with the development of palmistry. However, it is thought to have been heavily influenced by early Vedic culture,[2] with elements of this science found in the likes of *Shat Sāmudrika Shāstra*, a study that concerns itself with signs and symbols written upon the body.[3] Nowhere were these signs taken with more seriousness than those written upon the palm, hands (after all) being the appendage most likely to feature in the success or downfall of an individual.

Hastā Sanjivan, or 'portraits of the living hand', are often grouped into a number of categories such as those present from birth, those developed with age and, finally, inherited lines from injury, mutilation or bad posture. One of the earliest and most important categories of sign interpretation was that arising from the decipherment of birthmarks or lines taking the form of auspicious/inauspicious objects. One example of auspiciousness might be Padma (a lotus flower), identified with purity, compassion and clarity of mind. Conversely, Sarpa (snakes) were commonly identified with strife, hidden dangers or an uncertain future and so considered unlucky.

REKHAS (LINES)

Unlike the fixedness of a horoscope, lines upon the palm appeared subject to development, at times appearing, merging or fading. Lines were thought to coalesce or disburse as one accrued or discharged karmic debts. A detailed cataloguing of your own palm, over a period of years, often reveals an almost imperceptible shifting of secondary and miscellaneous lines. Primary lines such as life (Āyu), head (Matru), heart (Hṛdaya) and fate (karma) appear less subject to change, as these constitute the foundation stones of life, and as such are unlikely to be modified to any great extent. That being said, smaller tributaries or branches, feeding into or away from these primary lines, may be greatly influenced with the passing of years.

Lines on the palm begin to assert themselves more fully from around the age of twelve years.[4] A child's palm often appears simplistic or shallow in contrast to those of young adults or the furrowed, darkened adult examples. Some individuals bear few lines but those visible have both depth and gravity, appearing to drain or dwarf subsidiary lines. Other palms may show bewildering dendritic patterns, with no one line appearing to stand apart from its comrades. Overly simplistic examples like these may reflect how an individual feels their life to unfold, that is, the former feeling swept downstream with little chance to react, seemingly driven to a focal point, while the latter experiences constant side-tracking and detours, which eventually seem to return them to a similar set of circumstances.

OVERVIEW OF THE BOOK

Palmistry forms an important branch of India's predictive sciences, its volume and wealth of knowledge remaining vast. Throughout the pages of this book I have tried to distil its quintessential factors into something both practical and informative for the reader. Vedic Palmistry is here presented in five 'bite-size' partitions that are best considered pieces of a delicate puzzle that stand alone or if taken in totality lock neatly together, helping to cognise the subject's importance. As the number '5' is symbolic of the totality of fingers + thumb (on a hand), and 5 is the numeral most associated with occult sciences, its use here seems most appropriate.

Part I discusses the topography of the hand, along with a brief introduction to Āyurvedic[5] concepts of health, vitality and constitutional typing. This section also considers the three primary states of matter, known as *Gunas*, identifying their varying locations on palm and fingers.

Part II shows how the lines (Rekhas) can take the form of complex symbols, be conjoined or stand alone. Here we examine their numerous manifestations and interpretations, along with fingerprints (*Hastā-mudrā*) and timelines (Kālamāna Rekha), the latter offering a means to judge their manifestation.

Part III looks at the planets (Grahas) and zodiac signs (Rashis) as revealed upon the palm and fingers. Correlations between planets, zodiac signs and the individual are paramount to any understanding of palmistry. This section introduces each planet through a series of portraits, their significations, temperaments, mounds (on the palm) and associated lines.

Part IV covers the Nakshatras on the palm and fingers. Often referred to as lunar mansions, Nakshatras support any analysis of lines. Understanding their significations and propitiatory acts is considered key to placating or empowering the lines inscribed upon our palms.

Part V investigates prescribed methods of planetary appeasement. This very traditional component of Hastā Rekha (and Jyotish) aims to counteract (negative) or enhance (positive) planetary forces through the use of mantra, yantra, gemstones, among others.

NOTES

1. Palmistry, in the ancient world, may have been the preferred method of analysis by astrologers, having instant access to all planetary influences conveniently placed in the palm of the hand.
2. There remains conjecture over the true origins of this tradition, with Samudra Rishi believed to have compiled one of the earliest treaties on Sâmudrikam including Hastā Rekha Shāstra.
3. *Shat Sāmudrika Shāstra*: date, author and true origination remain unclear. Other references (in antiquity) to the practice of palmistry occur in Purāṇic texts such as *Vāyu Purāṇa* (Chapter LVII), *Garuda Purāṇa* (Chapter LXV) and *Agnī Purāṇa* (Chapter CCXLII), as well as *Brihat Saṃhitā* (Chapter LXVIII), authored by the esteemed astrologer and astronomer Varāhamihira. Additionally, 'tenuous' references to hand and fate are found in *Rig Veda* (Hymn CVXII) and *Atharva Veda Saṃhitā* VII 52.8.
4. Increments of 12 years are considered important junctures in Hastā Rekha; the all-important number 6 (6×2=12) has potent numerological significance in this science.
5. Āyurveda is a medicine system with historical roots firmly buried in the Indian subcontinent. There is no agreed date for its emergence; however, many believe it to be a concise health care system with a written history of some three thousand years. If its oral traditions are also considered, this date might be pushed back to a date of 5000 BC.

PART I

TOPOGRAPHY OF THE HAND

Chapter 1

WHICH HAND DO I LOOK AT?

There is some level of controversy over which hand should take precedence during palm analysis. Which hand represents what – and how to judge with factors such as gender, career and preference in use. The following provides five popular answers to this question:

- More ancient sources advise the right hand of a male is preferred during analysis, with the opposite being true of women. A man's left hand is considered his cast lot from birth, his right hand bearing those Rekha most likely to have been 'modified' by sustained effort/work (or the lack of it). The reverse is held to be true for a woman.
- The left hand is inscribed by that which has already passed (previous incarnation/karmas). Upon the right hand are those events which are current or yet to be. In short, each palm is unique to these expressions. This is true for either male or female.
- The hand that dominates, that is, leads by action or is steadiest, is to be preferred in analysis. That is to say, the hand by which an individual makes their livelihood. Rekha in this hand are most likely to affect the future.*
- Rekha seen in both hands are to be taken into due consideration, similar patterning taken as confirmation of fate. Where Rekha are divergent, the dominant hand should be taken to provide a final analysis.
- If a person is ambidextrous (preferring neither hand in daily tasks), the hand which bears the greatest profusion or depth of line is to be preferred.

* Throughout this book I will adhere to this third method, my instructor's preferred method of analysis (see Appendix for more information).

Chapter 2

HAND TOPOGRAPHY AND ĀYURVEDA

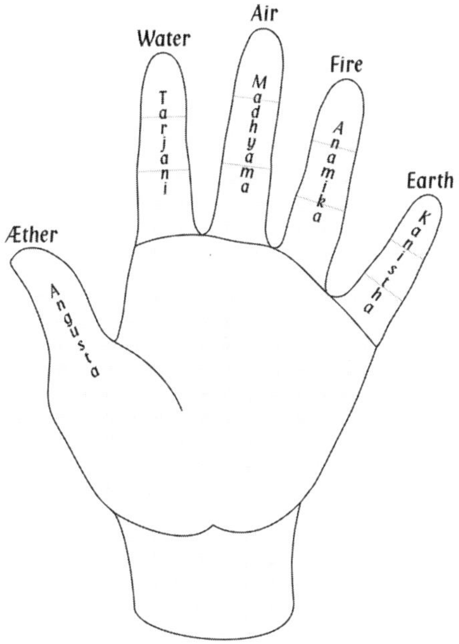

Key: Angusta = thumb, Tarjani = forefinger, Madhyama = middle finger, Anamika = ring finger and Kanistha = little finger. The five states of matter, or Pañca Mahabhuta, are represented by thumb/æther, forefinger/water, middle/air, ring/fire and little finger/earth.

According to some Āyurvedic sources, Sushruta[1] is thought to have said: 'Human hands are truly greatest amongst all tools, for they are the means by which all tools are fashioned.' Having such emphasis placed upon the hands, it seems only natural they should find themselves central to ancient practices of divination.

Vedic Palmistry identifies the four fingers and thumb as corresponding to the five states of matter[2] (pañca mahabhuta), the five senses (buddhīndriyas[3]), the five sense organs (pañca jñanendriyani[4]) and the five actions (karmendriyas[5]). The four fingers and their associated mounds (parvata) relate to four of the nine planets. The five remaining planets are assigned various positions or *sthana* about the palm. Each of the three phalanges on the four fingers denotes one of twelve zodiacal signs (known as Rashis[6]), with the two hands being symbolic of consciousness (puruṣa) and latent matter (prakṛti). Two hands relate also to discharged karma and those karmas yet to unfold. Destiny (dharma) is to be read from the lines upon the palm or through the appearance of symbols (chinha), nested in amongst a profundity of these lines. The presence of the latter was deemed an auspicious sign (laksanya), awarded either to alleviate or to teach a valuable life lesson. Using Āyurvedic principles, hands are firstly decoded using the principle of dominant element and dosha.[7] The five elements and their corresponding dosha are:

Vāta = Air and Æther

Pitta = Fire

Kapha = Water and Earth

As elements and dosha are interrelated, the qualities of each become detectable on the hand. As hands are generally less subject to change on the body, their analysis becomes an ideal first-tier investigative tool.

AIR HAND

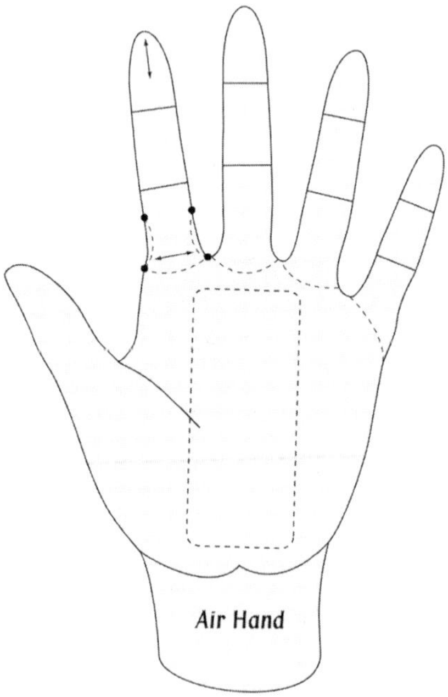

Air Hands have much in common with the Āyurvedic dosha Vāta (inclusive of æther).

Qualities of the Air Hand include dryness and coolness with delicate 'narrow' bone structuring and spatial irregularities of the phalanges. Often the distal phalanges appear ovular at the tip, while the fingers appear overly long[8] or short in relation to the length of the palm. For example, narrow palms will appear to accentuate finger length whereas long narrow palms will appear to shorten the finger length. Additionally, there may be a slight narrowing at the base of the proximal phalanges, while thumbs often appear long, wiry, dexterous and often double-jointed.

Overall, the Air Hand tends toward a rectangular form with slightly protruding joints. Rekha tend to be fine, profuse and branched, displaying multiple broken lines or cross-hatching. The nail beds are often dried, frayed and white. Nails are generally thin, brittle, chewed, lined or irregular looking; with an overall smoky whiteness. Typical traits of an Air Hand type include: dexterity, adaptability and an inherent distrust of authority figures. They are often verbally communicative, erratic, artistic, creative and slippery (hard to pin down). Though easily enthused, they are unable to sustain any long-term plan, often subject to mental fatigue or periodic physical exhaustion.

FIRE HAND

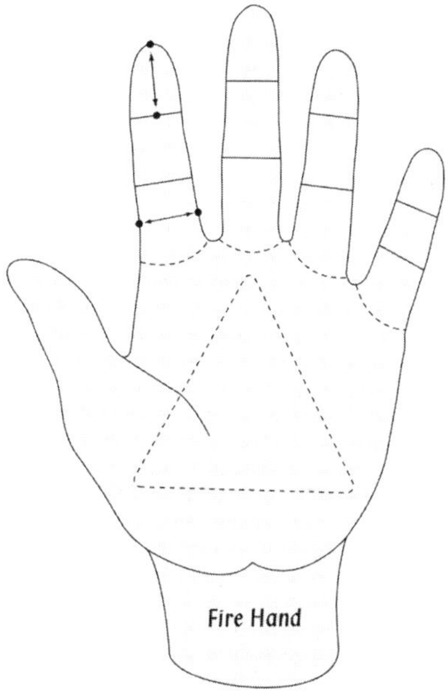

Fire Hands have much in common with the Āyurvedic dosha Pitta.

Qualities of the Fire Hand include warmth, smoothness (usually padded and shiny) with colourful blotches, redness, freckles and so on. Fingers are of medium length with little variation in width[9] except close to the lower proximal phalanges. The palm of the Fire Hand often shows a subdued triangular quality, its natural contours revealing a subtle triangular depression when fingers and thumb are brought together. Rekha tend to be well-defined, of medium depth but display a good number of reddened crosses or forks at the ends of primary lines. Keerthi Rekha may be present (ring finger/fire element) or strong Rekha present upon Kuja-sthana[10] displaying prominence or heightened colouration.

Nail beds are often raised, pink and prone to inflammation. Nails are of average thickness, slightly soft, tear easily or have a notable transparency (looking pinkish). Length of nails is often restricted due to their inherent softness. Traits of a Fire Hand type include: sharpness and stinginess, overly analytical, detail-orientated, dictatorial, opinionated, intellectually driven, easily provoked or angered, competitive, combative – yet philanthropic.

WATER HAND

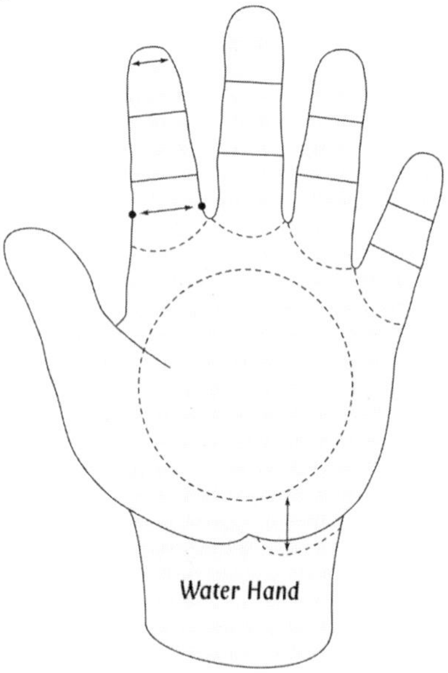

Water Hands have much in common with the Āyurvedic dosha Kapha (inclusive of earth).

Qualities of the Water Hand include strength, firmness and compactness with robust bone structuring and little spatial irregularity of phalanges. Often the distal phalange appears squared at the tip, while fingers may appear short in relation to the palm. Additionally, there may be a widening at the base of the proximal phalanges; thumbs are usually fleshy, stocky and strong – but can lack flexibility. The index finger (water element) may display prominent Rekha such as Guru Chandrika or Dīksha Rekha, fingertips may also appear spatulate (splayed). Chandra-sthana (moon's mound) may be elongated, exerting a watery influence on the constitution.

Overall, a Water Hand tends toward the circular or rounded form, masking the joints. Rekha are fewer in number but defined[11] showing fewer breaks but strongly rooted. Nail beds are wide, smooth (lubricated) and of a dense white composition. Nails are generally thick, smooth and regular, growing to a squared end. Water Hand types are often methodical and patient with an inherent distrust of the new; their actions speak louder than their words. They tend to be steady, sentimental and reliable with good long-term memories, conservative yet productive, unlikely to tire easily or abandon their course of action.

MIXED TYPES

Identifying predominant elements in a hand is a little like playing detective, sleuthing over topography, looking for clues before finally pulling it all together. In the real world, the three aforementioned pure types are somewhat of a rarity, most hands being a mixture of at least two predominating elements (with the third often following closely behind). For physical functionality to occur, all three dosha must be present; however, the precise composition of each individual is founded upon a very specific ratio of dosha known as *Prakṛuti*.[12] This mixture is allocated during conception and later imprinted on the physical and mental structure during the pregnancy term; this then becomes their core nature throughout life. If this mixture of dosha becomes imbalanced and left unchecked it will eventually accumulate to the point of becoming dominant and disruptive, taking its toll upon the individual. This latter principle is known as *Vikṛuti* or state of current imbalance. Ascertaining core-nature from a currently imbalanced state requires some specialist Āyurvedic skills; however, in the case of the hand its general appearance is unlikely to radically alter to a point where constitutional analysis becomes indeterminate or impossible. Hand identification and Rekha significations are often an ideal way to start evaluating constitution and karma. Table 2.1 represents a few guidelines for the identification of mixed hand types.

Table 2.1 Guidelines for the identification of mixed hand types

Air + Water	Air + Fire	Fire + Water
Medium build, cool and moist, pale/ashy in colouration, thicker nails	Medium to elongated, warm and dry, slight narrowing at the base of fingers	Medium to rounded build, soft fleshy fingers with squared tips, cool but reddish patches

Chapter 3

MAHA GUNA (SATTVA-RAJAS-TAMAS)

The three doshas, Vāta, Pitta and Kapha, are the cause of all pathology in the physical body. The gunas Rajas and Tamas are the cause of all pathology in the mind.

Caraka Saṃhitā

According to Sāṁkhya[13] (an ancient system of Indian philosophy), a dualistic interplay of primal forces called *puruṣa* (spirit/masculine) and *prakṛti* (matter/feminine) literally interweave the substance of the universe. Puruṣa might be likened to consciousness (devoid of matter), while prakṛti represents inert primal matter (devoid of consciousness). The former might be the considered masculine 'causal' principle, while the latter enacts a feminine 'creative' role. Once infused with consciousness/awareness, matter begins to move, bind and develop, gaining in momentum and complexity. This playground of matter becomes the medium through which all physical experience becomes possible.

Prakṛti is three-natured, or a composition of three qualities, each entwined about the others, like the strands of a rope. Collectively, these are referred to as *maha-guna*, individually referred to as *Sattva*, *Rajas* and *Tamas*. Energetically these three might be thought of as:

Sattva = virtuous, light and upward moving
Rajas = restless, turbulent and outward moving
Tamas = darkness, decay, heaviness and inertia

Sāṁkhya-Kārikā[14] likens the nature of the three guna to pleasure (prīti), pain (aprīti) and delusion (viṣāda). Their individual natures are said to illuminate, activate and fix. Ancient medical treatises such as *Sushruta Saṃhitā*[15] and *Aṣṭāñga Hṛdayam*[16] provide detailed and enlightening commentaries on the attributes of guna, saying:

- *Features of Sattva include:* persons of good conduct and moral behaviour, having clean habits, reading constantly from the Vedas, holding belief in a higher power and having reverence for their preceptors (elders). They are hospitable and celebrate, becoming involved with all religious festivals and sacrifices.

- *Features of Rajas include:* persons of affluent circumstance, valorous and irascible, gluttonous (fond of eating) – without sharing, they are talkative and vain. Angry and prideful, they are jealous of other men's excellence.
- *Features of Tamas include:* persons of parsimoniousness, perverse intellect and fearful, in whom frequent sexual dreaming occurs. Lazy and grief-stuck, they display the incapacity to determine truth from falsehood.

As with many classical texts, its language comes over as harsh and uncompromising to modern ears, but I also think the reader comes away with a fairly clear picture of their qualities. That being said, some 'positive' factors of each guna remain less highlighted. For instance, while sattvic encourages matter to evolve and rarefy, Tamas brings stability and durability (resistance), an essential quality required by organic matter to survive in hostile environments, Likewise, Rajas provides the impetus to move outward, explore and compete in those same hostile environments.

MAHA GUNA ON THE HAND

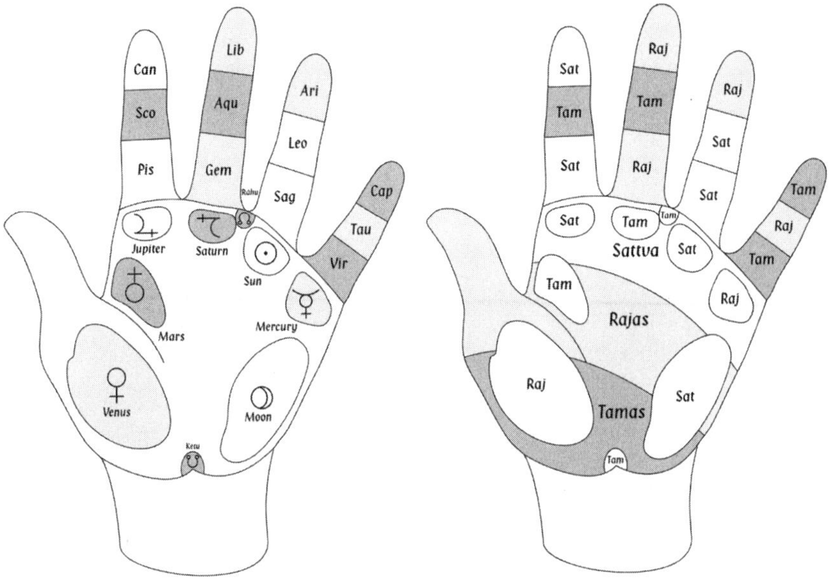

Planets and signs (left) with corresponding guna (right) as identified upon the hand.
Note: Positions are mirrored on both hands. Key: Sat = Sattva, Raj = Rajas and Tam = Tamas.

Maha Guna are read on the palm in a number of ways. First, the hand itself is separated into two parts: palm and fingers. The four fingers are apportioned amongst the 12 zodiacal signs and their allotted guna (see Part III for a detailed account of zodiacal signs). Then, the palm itself is divided into three: upper, middle and lower (see left diagram above). Accordingly, the higher zone is awarded Sattva qualities, the middle Rajas, and the lower palm Tamas. Lastly, the locations of planetary mounds (known as parvata; see Chapter 6) are accorded guna status, on the basis of their ruling planetary lord, these being as listed in Table 3.1. For a detailed account of planetary traits see Part III.

Table 3.1 The ruling planetary lords for the gunas

Sattva	Rajas	Tamas
Sun, Moon and Jupiter	Mercury and Venus	Mars, Saturn, Rāhu and Ketu

With regard to Maha Guna and the palm, it can seem a little contradictory or confusing to have a planetary mound governed by Sattva located in a tamasic zone. In instances such as these it should be kept in mind that planets, lines and symbols take precedence in palm analysis. So, for instance, an important symbol seen on the mound of Saturn would firstly be accorded tamasic qualities, even if located in the upper (sattvic) part of the palm. Similarly, lines resting on the mound of the Moon would be accorded sattvic qualities, even when located in the lower tamasic part of the palm. Maha Guna do add an extra dimension to any analysis, but their influence should not override the primary effects of planets, lines and symbols.

NOTES

1. Originator of *Susrutha Saṃhitā*, a treatise in Sanskrit on surgical techniques and internal medicine c.100 BCE–200 BCE.
2. Space (æther), movement (air), transformation (fire), humidity (water) and cohesion (earth).
3. Sight, hearing, smell, taste and touch.
4. Ears, skin, eyes, tongue and nose.
5. Speaking, grasping, walking, elimination and sexual pleasure.
6. Distribution of the five elements in accordance with elements awarded to each sign; for example, Cancer, Scorpio and Pisces (water signs) are located on the index or water element finger. Symbolically, the thumb (æther element) provides containment (and is contained) within of all elements. As such, a thumb may comfortably rest (over) or be covered by (under) the four fingers.
7. There is no direct translation of dosha; however, 'defect' is often used. Each dosha therefore presents itself as the means by which the individual is most likely to succumb to dis-ease by its accumulation, resulting in metabolic imbalances.
8. This is especially true of the middle finger, being Saturn ruled and also representing the air element.
9. The index finger is often proportionally wider than the remaining fingers.
10. Kuja = Mars, Sthana = position. For more information on planetary positions see 'Planetary Mounds' in Chapter 6.
11. Definition comes from depth rather than colouration.
12. Prakṛuti = first nature.
13. Sāṁkhya Philosophy is mostly credited to the sage Kapila. Although mentioned in *Rigveda*, his era remains unclear. Sāṁkhya means the science of enumeration, listing the basic principles of existence as numbering 24. Sāṁkhya Philosophy also underpins the Āyurvedic Philosophy.
14. One of the oldest surviving texts on Saṁkhya philosophy, exact date unknown. Chinese translations became available toward the end of the sixth century AD.
15. *Sārīrasthāna* Chapter IV.
16. *Sārīrasthāna* Chapter III.

PART II

THE LINES (REKHAS)

Chapter 4

REKHAS (LINES)

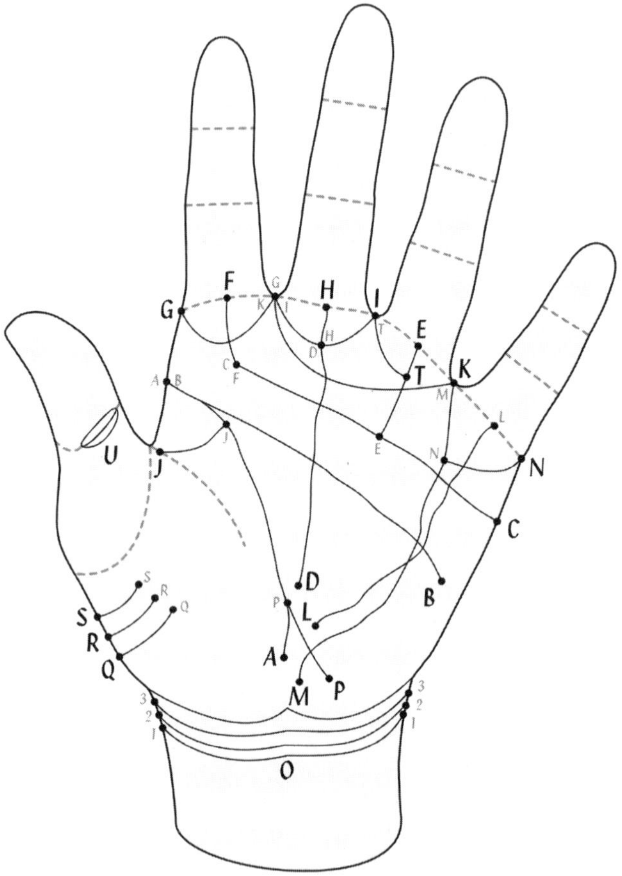

Primary Lines: (A) Life Line/Āyu Rekha, (B) Head Line/Matru Rekha, (C) Heart Line/Hṛdaya Rekha, (D) Fate Line/Karma Rekha. Secondary Lines: (E) Sun Line/Keerthi Rekha, (F) Jupiter Line/Dīksha Rekha, (G) Jupiter Crescent/Guru Chandrika, (H) Saturn Line/Shani Rekha, (I) Saturn Crescent/ Shani Chandrika, (J) Line of Enemies/Maṅgal Rekha, (K) Venus Belt/Shukra Mekhala, (L) Contentment Line/Sukha Rekha, (M) Mercury Line/Budh Rekha, (N) Union Line/ Vivāha Rekha, (O) Bracelets/Maṇibandha Rekha, (P) Moon Line/Chandra Rekha, (Q) Progeny Line/Sāntana Rekha, (R) Siblings Line/Bhartr Rekha, (S) Kinship Line/ Bhaṇḍu Rekha, (T) Fortune Line/Punya Rekha, (U) Thumb Barley/Anguśta Mula Yava.

The lines on the palm form a connective bridge between planetary mounds and symbols. These dendritic branches intertwine across the palm to produce an individual's signature of vitality,[1] wealth and longevity. Much as inscriptions upon the face of yantra resonate with its desired effect, so too do the lines appropriate and direct planetary emissions – toward whatever ends an individual's karma calls for.

Indian palmistry divides lines intro three distinct categories: Primary (Pradhāna), Secondary (Aṃśāṃśa) and Miscellaneous (Prakīrṇa). Most if not all individuals display some semblance of the four primary lines, although some may appear dominant or recessive in comparison to their companion lines. There are cases when the two Primary transversal lines (Heart and Head) intertwine, appearing singular. Such patterning is sometimes termed Markaṭa Rekha (ape line), this configuration commonly seen upon the hands of simians. Hastā Rekha may defer to this rather derogatory term when referring to a single crease traversing the centre of the palm. This combination of primary Rekha is said to heighten wilful and stubborn characteristics, driving individuals toward obsessive self-preservation and self-gratification.

Although not to be considered exhaustive, the following provides a general overview of the lines and their interpretation.

PRIMARY LINES (PRADHĀNA)

- *Life Line[2] (Āyu/Pitru[3] Rekha[4]):* Perhaps the most infamous of all lines extends from under or upon the mound of Jupiter, curving about the thumb downward toward the wrist and bracelets. The Life Line separates two zones upon the palm, that is, comfort and material needs, as defined by the mounds of Venus and Mars in opposition to the remaining planets: Saturn (suffering), Sun (fame), Mercury (intellect) and Moon (emotion). Ideally Life Lines should be long, deep and of good colouration, without breaks or chaining (see 'Miscellaneous Lines (Prakīrṇa)'). The Life Line is thought to represent the paternal blood-line, that is, strengths and weaknesses derived from the father. This line also describes the individual's relationship toward their father, or to their perception of the father's ability (or inability) to manifest in the material world. Life Lines have been described as the primary significator of vitality (prāna) and life-span; however, when judging longevity this line must always be considered in conjunction with the Fate Line, Mercury Line (if present) and the bracelets seen at the wrist. A Life Line commencing with strong roots promotes stability, wisdom and longevity; it may also indicate those afforded much support during their formative years or those in whom a keen interest in history has or will develop. Chained, poorly rooted or broken beginnings to this line indicate a less than favourable start in life, also leaving an individual less likely to receive support during their life-time. It may also indicate an individual lacking in discipline or one who becomes easily disorientated/diffused with regard to their own ambitions or goals.

- *Head Line (Matru[5] Rekha):* This is studied to ascertain the strength of the individual's maternal blood-line. This line also indicates the individual's mental state as well as the physical condition of the head and brain. The Head Line additionally encompasses self-confidence, self-awareness, long-term memory and mental health. The Head and Life Lines share a point of common origination, providing a snapshot of early parental influence. Their point of separation identifies the individual's breaking point with group identity and the establishment of self-awareness, that is, a sense of personal mortality. For more information about the timing of this event see the section 'Timelines (Kālamāna Rekha)' at the end of this chapter. Head Lines should usually follow a gentle downward curve, toward the mound of the Moon. This is also an area of mind, emotion and imagination; indeed, termination of any Primary Line in this area is an indicator for heightened dexterity, creative skills (artistic temperament) or nervous anxiety. The more acute the angle between Head and Life Lines, the deeper the Head Line is driven onto the mound of the Moon. A deeply furrowed Head Line, ending well inside the lunar area, indicates those who are highly impressionable or very abstract in thought. The individual may also be subject to periodic cycles of depression. Head Lines terminating in a fork or at a crossing line on the mound of the Moon should be carefully assessed to determine the dominant fork. If the overall trend is downward pointing toward ever greater lunar dominance, the individual may become highly capricious, self-obsessed or engage in hypochondria. An upward turning fork toward the mound of Mercury suppresses these self-indulgent tendencies and emotive outbursts, steering the individual toward inward and objective self-analysis.
- *Heart Line (Hṛdaya Rekha):* This emanates from the base of the little finger (below the mound of Mercury), upwardly traversing the palm toward Jupiter's mound and the index finger. Heart Lines determine the individual's health and wellbeing. This line promotes courage,

strength and our ability to love or be loved. It also promotes self-healing and/or the will to overcome adversity. On a physical level, this line represents the heart, blood and nervous system, also indicating our rate of recovery from injury, illnesses or trauma. The Heart Line is deemed optimal when deeply rooted under the mound of Mercury. It should be rich in colour, even in width and unbroken. It should follow an unbroken course toward the base of the index finger. If faint, chained or overly inflicted by crossing or radiating lines from Saturn's mound, the Heart Line becomes disturbed, weakened or of low morale. This line is almost always traversed by the Fate Line and so should be carefully examined to determine which path takes precedence. When the Heart Line dominates the Fate Line and continues unabated, the individual prospers, gaining recognition, wealth and respectability. If the Fate Line dominates the Heart Line, the individual may suffer physically through guilt, depression or blame; yet may still achieve some position of authority or influence in the world.

- *Fate Line (Karma Rekha[6]):* It is said that even those born of noble character, education and excellence will be unable to receive reward without the blessing of destiny. This rather ominous line (with strong Saturnine overtones) is more often than not aligned centrally upon the palm, cleaving it vertically. The base of this line is usually entwined about the home of Ketu (the southern lunar node; see Chapter 6), its terminus falling upon the mound of Saturn. Strong, deep destiny lines, emanating from the lower palm, are thought to protect health, promote digestive strength[7] and project a strong character. Those with a strong Fate Line appear firmly entrenched upon their life-path. If this line appears faint, crooked or chained it denotes a changeable character or greater uncertainty surrounding the individual's fate. Broken or missing sections of line can indicate short periods of relationship intensity, financial setback or multiple career instabilities. Islands and chaining (see the section 'Miscellaneous Lines (Prakīrṇa)') often indicate depressive bouts, low immunity or the inability to assimilate vital minerals. If the Fate Line terminates upon contacting the Head Line, an individual may break with family traditions or seek a career beyond their social caste. Generally, Fate Lines are considered auspicious if appearing to display an upward motion (or urdhwa), proceeding unbounded toward the mound of Saturn. Well-defined and unbroken, the Fate Line lessens uncertainty or setback. As with any palm analysis, supporting lines should also be taken into account, for instance an individual bearing *anurekha* (support line; see the section 'Miscellaneous Lines (Prakīrṇa)') or *chatuśkōṇa* (squares; see the section 'Miscellaneous Lines (Prakīrṇa)') are more likely to mitigate the potential negativity of a poorly disposed Fate Line.

SECONDARY LINES (AṂŚĀṂŚA)

Of no less importance, these when present are:

- *Sun Line (Keerthi Rekha):* This is considered a blessed line, its presence said to impart radiance, making an individual stand out. This line promotes intelligence and success in all undertakings, earning the individual admiration from his/her peers. A Sun Line gives unexpected career opportunity or promotion, and may also place the individual under the tutelage or protective wing of a renowned master. It can also signify those engaged in the political arena, or philanthropic endeavours. While a Sun line can soften the personality, those bearing its mark are not to be trifled with, very often having impeccable connections and powerful friends.
- *Jupiter Line (Dīksha Rekha):* This is an auspicious yet infrequently seen line promoting intelligence, wisdom, confidence, optimism and patience. The presence of a Jupiter Line guides one toward centres of learning and education in a quest for higher knowledge. Its presence also denotes those apprenticed with a master of some renown. The blessing of this line is said to secure the wellbeing of one's progeny as well as seeing a positive return on any investment (children being our greatest investment!). On a slightly negative note, Jupiter Lines can also incline one toward arrogance, over-indulgence or over-expansion – literally, gluttony.
- *Jupiter Ring[8] (Guru Chandrika[9]):* This produces similar results to the Jupiter Line, with a greater emphasis on intense levels of research and study, particularly those that ultimately benefit society as a whole. A ring surrounding the mound of Jupiter is often linked to craftsmen, lawyers, adjudicators or those preferring lives of tranquillity and seclusion. It may also be found on those who pursue teaching careers. Partially complete rings signify a tendency to start studies in earnest, only to switch their efforts at a later date. Lines intersecting any ring should also be considered, their ultimate source discovered and considered. Intersecting lines to this ring usually denote interference or insecurities.

- *Saturn Line (Shani Rekha):* Generally a positive line; however, it can unduly burden a individual with worry and over-responsibility. Care should be taken to ascertain if this line is distinct from the Fate Line or merely its extension onto the mound of Saturn. An authentic Saturn Line should be separate from the Fate Line. A Saturn Line promotes endurance, longevity and health; those bearing this line attain positions of authority, aided and abetted by loyal friends. This line also promises a modest accumulation of wealth, although returns tend to be through long-term investment. When weakened or afflicted, this line may indicate accidents, injury or chronic long-term sicknesses.

- *Saturn Ring (Shani Chandrika[10]):* This produces similar results to a Saturn Line except that the individual acquires a greater interest in spiritual matters, perhaps through some form of spiritual practice (known as sādhanā[11]). The ring of Saturn is considered an auspicious mark yet is somewhat of a rarity. Its presence suggests a life of renunciation, retreating into nature and/or solitude. When other elements support these inclinations (see Part III) the individual generally finds a way to integrate some form of asceticism into their lives. If more worldly signs are present (such as a Venus Belt or Mercury Line), the transition to a spiritual path can be more complicated and painful. Those bearing this ring often have some strong inner faith or are drawn toward religions such as Hinduism, Jainism or Buddhism, all of which embrace renunciation. Those carrying this mark may also take great benefit from the worship of Lord Śiva.

- *Mars Line (Maṅgala Rekha[12]):* This line generally foments enmity, physical altercations, scars, anger, violence or injustice. All of these might be directed toward the individual (particularly during their youth[13]). The proximity of this line to the Life Line heavily impacts longevity, usually by increasing fire (Pitta dosha; see Chapter 2) – that is, fevers, inflammation or blood impurities. The impact of this line is most likely to damage the heart, liver, gallbladder or spleen.[14] On a positive note, a Mars Line can increase vitality, courage and fortitude, its presence a clear indication of some enhanced élan-vital. If straight, clean and well-defined, a Mars Line can presage an active life with little incidence of disease (all other factors considered). This line may also indicate a proclivity for any Martian skill such as athletics (sports), surgery, acupuncture, metal-working or alchemy.

- *Venus Belt (Shukra Mekhala):* This is one of the most commonly seen secondary lines and easily identified as its girth embraces the mounds of the Sun and Saturn. It is interpreted largely by its fullness or distance from the base of ring and middle fingers. When positioned close to the Heart Line, a Venus Belt assumes greater positivity; that is, the individual develops an affectionate disposition, is attracted to the arts (performing, visual or literary), attains great successes or is simply fond of the opposite sex. When the line is broken, drawn close toward the base of ring and middle finger or when mirrored by supporting lines,[15] the individual can develop an unhealthy obsession with sex. They may also endure much hardship in relationships or frequently change their partner – becoming easily dissatisfied in matters of love.

- *Contentment Line (Sukha Rekha):* Sometimes described as an additional Health Line (after a Mercury Line), its presence is overall considered benign. Contentment Lines promote a healing ability or a deeper interest in matters of health and longevity. Any negative connotations of this line include self-obsession (hypochondria) or addictions. To be a true Contentment Line it must be independent of a Mercury Line. A Contentment Line may be classified as anurekha (major support line); if seen, it is usually equal in length to the Mercury Line.

- *Mercury Line (Budha Rekha):* This is also known as a health, intuition or business line. When present, this line may give mixed results, but for the most part is seen as having a positive influence. Emanating from the middle of the lower palm, usually at the edge of the mound of the Moon, it moves upward toward the mound of Mercury, clipping the mound of the Moon to varying degrees. Its point of termination is usually on the mound of Mercury or close to the base of the little finger. Mercury Lines are renowned for giving business acumen or an urge to travel. They may also signify healing potential; that is, they are thought to promote healing abilities. Renowned for agility and speed of communication, Mercury Lines may also imbue the individual with precognitive abilities (forecasting future events with some accuracy); they may also have an uncanny knack of predicting financial markets, making them healthy returns on wise investments. Those bearing this line often back the right horse or decline business ventures (later to fail), hence this line is also known as *the line of intuition*. Any negativity connected to this line usually manifests as hypochondria, skin conditions or an overly sensitive digestive tract. The individual may also become flighty, fidgety, unable to stick to any single course of action. Mercury Lines may also make one prone to bouts of low immunity, often brought on through overwork or mental fatigue.

- *Union Line (Vivāha[16]):* Usually seen on the upper percussion of the hand, running horizontally, across the mound of Mercury, its presence denotes a warm and affectionate character. It also manifests as the need to nourish or defend those cast aside. This line is considered to give feminine qualities to its bearer. A strong Union Line here indicates the desire for long-term relationships or commitment. It may also suggest a character needing to be cared for. The Union Line has some impact on health and longevity due to its proximity to Heart and Mercury Lines as a union or partnership always brings some degree of change into daily routines. Such changes include diet, sleep patterns and stresses associated with co-habitation. All of these have a profound impact on health – for better or worse.
- *Bracelets (Maṇibandha Rekha[17]):* These are located at the edge of the lower palm and wrist. Bracelets are a book in their own right as much controversy surrounds their true import or interpretation. The word maṇibandha means fixed jewel (maṇi = jewel and bhandha = to fix) and wrists have always been associated with the wearing of amulets (protective jewellery). This gave rise to the interpretation of bracelets as foundations or protectorates of the palm.[18] Bracelets have long been regarded as the three pillars of life –that is, wealth (dhana), knowledge (shāstra) and devotion (bhakti) – and move from lowest (toward elbow) to highest (toward fingertip). Although three lines are commonly seen, as many as six lines can be present, though it is unlikely that all are well-defined. Under normal circumstances bracelets represent three timelines, totalling sixty years (3×20 years). (See the section 'Timelines (Kālamāna Rekha)' at the end of this chapter for more information.) The most prominent bracelet takes precedence, highlighting that area in which the greater amount of life-force will be expended and during which time period that is likely to occur, that is, childhood, adulthood or old age (again counted upward toward the palm). Bracelets, if indistinct, pale, broken or chained, weaken the constitution. The more bracelets are affected, the more delicate the constitution. Weakened bracelets invariably lead to lowered immunity. In the absence of multiple bracelets, all transversal lines close to the edge of the lower palm are to be considered a type of bracelet, particularly if its route brings

it into close contact with the house of Ketu.[19] The transition of bracelets across the wrist reflects the individual's life-journey and general experiences, that is, true, clear and defined or convoluted, diluted and indistinct.

- *Moon Line (Chandra Rekha):* Deemed a mixed blessing, Moon Line's latitude should be carefully assessed. If resident in the top third of the Moon mound it produces results comparable to Sun Lines, promoting longevity, luck, fame and fortune through self-effort.[20] The individual may also feel the need to reinvent themselves with some regularity, to feel popular. Moon Lines found at the lower third of the Moon mound can promote self-obsession (vanity), hypochondria or depression; however, this portion of the lunar mound is also known to bear fruit for those artistically inclined. Moon Lines found in the middle third of the lunar mound display mixed qualities of the aforementioned. Overall, indications for a Moon Line incline the individual to endure periods of emotional fatigue, but ultimately attain some order of wealth (albeit later in life). Those bearing this line seem destined to end their days residing in lands foreign to their place of birth.
- *Progeny Line (Santāna Rekha):* This is one of a number of lines seen climbing vertically on the lower part of the Venus mound (see also the lines of Siblings and Relatives). This line is usually read as progeny or the desire to procreate. When seen and well-defined (straight, vertical and richly coloured), it indicates that children are to be expected. The closer to the hand's percussion, the earlier in life children appear. Broken, faint or chained lines may indicate difficulties in childbirth such as miscarriages or abortions, or severe childhood illnesses. Multiple horizontal lines crossing the Offspring Line delay birth/s or create insecurity in the individual, giving rise to doubt or worry over support and care of children. The sequence of progeny and sex was once read along this line, from the percussion to the palm's centre; however, this technique appears to have been lost – although some still claim to be able to interpret its signs.
- *Sibling Line (Bhrātru Rekha):* Located adjacent the Progeny Line, a Sibling Line is taken to be the next prominent line in a trine, moving incrementally upward toward the base of the thumb. It is interpreted as one's relationship toward younger sibling/s. In the absence of any siblings, this line gauges camaraderie toward younger friends in whom one identifies a surrogate sibling. A strong Sibling Line

indicates powerful allies or those who rally to the individual's cry ('brothers in arms'). Its presence may also indicate the physical strength of one's siblings (or allies). Faint, broken or crossing lines indicate estranged or wounded ties to those one would call a sibling.

- *Kinship Line (Bhanḍu Rekha):* The final line in the aforementioned trine occupies the highest position, often seen feeding into the line between the mound of Venus and the base of the thumb. Kinship Lines are given over to elder brothers and sisters as well as near relatives. This line can also be read as a wealth line due to legacies or financial support forthcoming from elder siblings and relatives. A strong line here indicates established kin (financial and social), more than likely to support the individual. Faint, broken or crossing lines here indicate estranged or unsuccessful elder siblings/relatives, unlikely to form any significant ties or be overly supportive to the individual.
- *Fortune Line (Punya Rekha[21]):* This line is located at the base of the ring finger, curving away from the mound of Saturn in toward the Sun mound, joining a Sun Line (if present). When present, they are mutually supportive, having similar indications. The presence of either is considered highly auspicious. Both lines amplify the positive benefit of the Sun mound, spreading name and fame over great distances or adding weight (and authority) to one's words. The Fortune Line makes one successful in their chosen vocation, attaining merit for their skills. The appearance of this line bestows the blessings of Sarasvatī, goddess of knowledge, art, music and wisdom.
- *Thumb Barley (Anguśta Mula Yava):* Located on the middle phalange of the thumb, this line's appearance (if fully formed) bears a remarkable resemblance to a kernel of barley. When present, this line ensures that the individual does not go without sustenance. To the ancients, this was indeed a highly welcome and auspicious sign. Barley kernels on both thumbs proclaimed those likely to feed beyond their means. In today's society this might be interpreted as those who enjoy playing host, feeding all equally. Although this configuration is often witnessed on the juncture of many fingers, its presence on the thumb[22] was deemed to be its most auspicious placement.

MISCELLANEOUS LINES (PRAKĪRṆA)

These are breaks or shapes occurring in tandem with Primary or Secondary Lines.

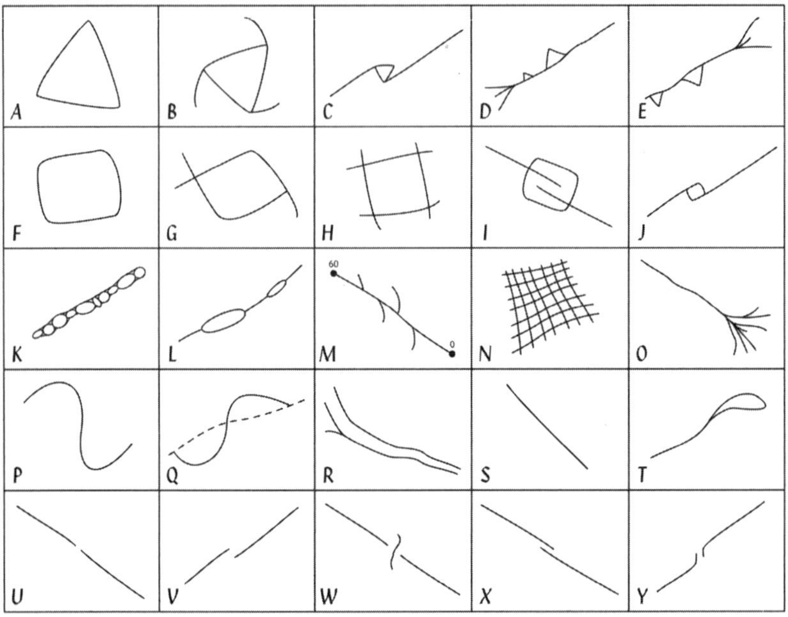

Miscellaneous Lines: (A) stand-alone triangles, (B) triangles with limbs, (C) healing triangles, (D) triangles above lines, (E) triangles below lines, (F) isolated squares, (G–H) limbed squares, (I) encapsulating squares, (J) healing squares, (K) chains, (L) islands, (M) support lines minor, (N) netting, (O) branched, (P) serpents, (Q) serpents as flags, (R) sister lines, (S) simple lines, (T) looped lines, (U) clean breaks, (V) broken lines without overlap, (W) crossing lines, (X) broken lines with overlap and (Y) hidden injury lines.

A. *Stand-alone triangles (Trikona)* are generally benefic and protective, their presence representing an opportunity to accumulate/benefit through invention, improvisation and decisive action. If found in close proximity to Primary Lines, their presence indicates an entrepreneurial talent, that is, likely to establish status, independent of others' wealth. Triangles located near or on the mound of Mars tend to attract litigation; however, one is likely to secure a beneficial outcome in disputes.

B. *Triangles with limbs* deliver success (fortune) with strings attached. This sign is generally benefic, but less so than its stand-alone counterparts.

C. *Healing triangles* bridging Primary or Secondary Lines denote accelerated healing or a patch/repair made to those lines. Their point of intersection (on Primary Lines or bracelets) may also be interpreted via timelines, that is, when this action is likely to be initiated.

D. *Triangles above lines* indicate financial gains; positioned below they indicate a wealth of knowledge or discovery.

E. *Triangles below lines*: see D.

F. *Isolated squares (Chatuśkōṇa)* are generally benefic, protecting line integrity by envelopment. These boxes may aid in the containment of disease/toxins, for example. Squares, having equal sides, represent sheltering or a metaphor for the body; their presence additionally indicates some level of internal healing as the body fights to isolate bodily systems and organs from external pathogens.

G. *Limbed squares* are a less auspicious variation, but still act in some healing capacity, albeit less efficiently.

H. *Limbed squares (variation)*: Here four independent lines unite, producing a square shape. The benefits of this configuration become solely dependent upon the quality of the lines forming its boundaries.

I. *Encapsulating squares.* Their presence suggests healing to lines over an extended period and may also indicate times of trauma or heightened stresses.

J. *Healing squares*, when positioned over broken lines, attempt to defend and strengthen. Their presence suggests an effort to remove the individual from harm's way. Their point of intersection and manifestation (on Primary Lines or bracelets) may be interpreted via timelines.

K. *Chains (Shrinḳhala)* are generally considered less favourable as chaining weakens all lines, unnecessarily confusing or diffusing strength. Chaining may also be indicative of delays, obstructions or heightened nervousness.

L. *Islands (Dweepa)*, when witnessed on Primary Lines, indicate difficulty, setbacks and delays during their respective time periods (see the section 'Timelines (Kālamāna Rekha)' at the end of this chapter). Islands also indicate periods of self-refection, changes in direction or re-evaluation of personal circumstances.

M. *Support lines minor (anurekha)* emanate directly from Primary or Secondary Lines. When appearing either side of a vertical Primary/ Secondary Line, anurekha strengthen and support. When seen above a horizontal Primary/Secondary line, they lift, strengthen and improve the vitality of that line; if seen below, the opposite effect may be expected.

N. *Netting*[23] *(Āvarita*[24]*)* indicates nervousness, hyperactivity or anxiety. Netting attached to a particular planetary mound traps (catches) the emissions of that planet, creates blockages. The more constrictive its weave, the greater its ability to restrict. Netting has been linked to cycles of depression, radical mood swings or areas of physical stagnation within the body. Planets or lines heavily encumbered by nets find it hard to get going, that is, gain momentum.

O. *Branched lines (Vijrumbhita)*, also referred to as 'roots', are commonly seen on the palm. Branches may occur on any line, at their point of origination or termination. Branches denote solid foundations and promote healthy lines. Branches also symbolise diversity, adaptability and fruition. The direction/position of the strongest limb determines its power source. Branches (in general) incline one toward writing, public service or research, their presence often manifesting as a strong interest in history or in ancient traditions. Overly intricate or indistinct branches may create confusion, indeterminacy or a loss of will-power.

P. *Serpents (Sarpa Rekha)* are generally inauspicious, their presence causing delays or periods of uncertainty. These lines may also be coupled with a loss of strength or resolve. If closely associated with the houses of Rāhu, Ketu or bracelets their negativity is somewhat reduced. In instances such as these, one will often travel or benefit from goods (or services) from overseas. If found in association with the Mercury Line, serpents create an interest in occult matters, such as palmistry and astrology. When found closely associated with the Fate Line, the individual may be forced to enter into litigation, although they will almost certainly be compensated for hardship or defamation of character.

Q. *Serpents as flags (Dwaja)* connected by their ends to the same line are interpreted as flags; see the next section, 'Symbols (Chinha)', for more information.

R. *Sister lines (anurekha)* run in tandem with other lines. The presence of this support line also strengthens and improves their companion, adding resistance and bridging weakened sections. Sister lines facilitate a temporary *jump-track*, offering a kind of fail-safe that runs unobtrusively in the background until needed. In a more negative aspect, Sister lines heighten sensitivity in their companion line. For example, conjoined with the Life Line, they may increase feelings of age, vulnerability or mortality. Conjoined with a Mercury Line they may promote nervous fatigue or hypochondria. Their presence may also indicate previous good merit (purva-punya), that is, areas where the individual excels without seeming to apply any effort.

S. *Simple lines (Sarala Rekha)* indicate events or actions sprung without prior warning. Although generally positive, simple lines may occur anywhere, appearing in isolation on the palm. Any or all benefits or losses obtained via these lines tend to be short-lived.

T. *Looped lines (Valitha Rekha)* are generally inauspicious, the presence of a loop at the end of a line indicating mental fatigue and instabilities. In some severe cases this may even lead to psychosis. Loops at the start of lines indicate false starts, loss of purpose or deception perpetrated by others.

U. *Clean breaks (Vi shrinḳhala)* are generally inauspicious. The presence of a broken line may indicate failure, or the inability to admit failure. All truncated lines denote insufficiency or inherent loss of energy along that line.

V. *Broken lines without overlap (Vi shrinḳhala)* indicate susceptibility to accidents or involvement in some kind of natural disaster. Traditionally these types of line were equated to injuries via one of the four great elements. For example: air/vāyu might equate to atmospheric disturbances; fire/tejas might equate to burns through incendiaries; water/jala could relate to floods or drowning; and earth/prithvi could relate to sinking or earthquakes. Ascertaining which element is causal requires identification of the planet or astrological sign most directly involved with that line.

W. *Crossing lines (Adhigamya Rekha)* display a thin space at their point of intersection. Crossing lines are generally considered inauspicious, especially in connection with a Primary Line; however, crossing lines on the palm are inevitable so their presence should not be looked upon with undue worry. Most instances of crossing are judged to foment delays, giving rise to frustration or temporary setbacks.

X. *Broken lines with overlap (Vi shrinkhala)* indicate an attempt to remedy long-overdue situations or injuries; however, they also indicate that healing remains temporary, returning to haunt one during their later years.

Y. *Hidden injuries line (Vi shrinkhala)* indicates hidden or secondary injuries incurred during a healing period. This type of line is generally inauspicious, noted to impair the healing of lines.

SYMBOLS (CHINHA)

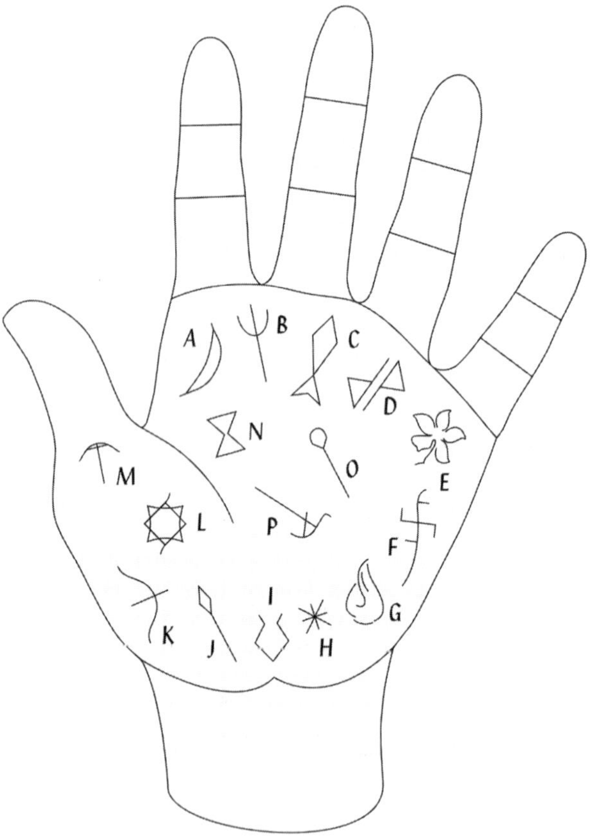

Auspicious symbols seen on the palm: (A) crescent moon, (B) trident, (C) fish, (D) flags, (E) lotus, (F) swastika, (G) conch, (H) six-pointed star, (I) water pot, (J) spear, (K) bow and arrow, (L) eight-pointed star, (M) umbrella, (N) two-headed drum, (O) mace and (P) plough.

Palms are also to be examined for Chinha (auspicious symbols)[25] – these can sometimes be overtly obvious or lurk deeper within other patterns. The general rule for a symbol is: the more distinguishable, the more assured its manifestation. Above all, the connection of each symbol to neighbouring lines provides the most valuable insights into its manifestation and timing (see 'Timelines (Kālamāna Rekha)' at the end of this chapter). In this section we explore a few popular (admittedly rare) symbols seen on the palm.

A. *Crescent Moon (Chandra):* May denote noble persons, those with a pronounced destiny or individuals likely to earn the affections of the public in general. A crescent moon denotes one enjoying the countenance of Lord Śiva, bestowing popularity,[26] longevity and beauty. This lunar symbol is thought to connect one to the healing arts, specifically through the medium of plants/herbs, elixirs and cooling waters. See also 'Moon Line' in the earlier section on 'Secondary Lines (Aṃśāṃśa)'.

B. *Trident (Trishula):* Traditionally taken to be an insignia of Shaivism,[27] the trident confers both religious and social honour, denoting those who are learned and wise. Tridents positioned close to (or upon) one of the Primary Lines indicate success in all ventures associated with that line. Tridents connected to the Fate Line delay one's introduction to their life-teacher (guru), forcing an individual to seek out many instructors. Seen in combination with the Life Line, a trident indicates the search for enlightenment through many disciplines, including those held to be socially unacceptable. Classical interpretation of tridents indicates those who are destined to be raised to great heights, acquiring fame and fortune – residing in the company of kings. If downward pointing, tridents are deemed less favourable, although still indicative of learned and wise individuals. Downward-facing tridents were thought to delay merit until earned, or force an individual to face slander for seeking fame at any cost.

C. *Fish (Matsya):* The presence of a fish was considered extremely lucky, offering protection from life's harder knocks. Fishes generally activate their associated planetary lords; for example, fish entwined about the Fate Line emphasise the role of Saturn in a positive way. This might manifest through promotion in career or gaining the loyalty and respect of co-workers or the acquisition of fixed assets. Associated with the Mercury Line, fishes improve health, healing or trading opportunities. When a fish appears to swim upwardly (toward the fingers), individuals acquire wealth and fame, but quickly gravitate toward material comforts. If facing downward (toward the wrist), an individual strives for deeper knowledge but attains little financial remuneration, or bequeaths any gain to philanthropic causes.

D. *Flag (Dwaja):* This is a symbol of distinction or one who makes their mark. Flags in close proximity to any of the Primary Lines promote notoriety and wealth. Directly associated with a planetary mound or planetary line, the merits of its lord become greatly enhanced. For example, associated with the Mercury Line, an individual gains recognition for their healing skills; associated with the mound of Mars, one becomes an outstanding athlete; with Rāhu, a renowned chemist. Upright flags (pointing toward fingers) promise social, political and financial advancement. Downward-pointing flags have similar effects but tend to slow the arrival of recognition, or to deliver merit when the individual least expects it. Flags also represent hidden wealth and its discovery in speculative markets. Individuals bearing this symbol are quite often found to prosper via investments connected to precious metals, gemstones and minerals.

E. *Lotus (Padma[28]):* This is a rare and auspicious symbol, denoting purity, compassion and clarity of mind. The symbol is said to be reserved for enlightened beings. Considered a blessing from Lord Brahmā, the lotus is renowned for its creationist symbolism as well as a deep connection to the primal elements *water* and *earth*. As the radiance of its flower bursts forth from the murky depths, so too do those who carry this symbol upon their palm, rising quickly from relative obscurity to become great leaders or inspirational figures.

F. *Spoked Cross (Swastika[29]):* Modern interpretations of this age-old occult symbol have mixed connotations; however, swastikas in India remain potent symbols, auspicious and full of talismanic properties. Those fortuitous enough to bear this mark on their palm are believed to be 'watched over', destined become powerful figures, attaining notoriety for outspoken viewpoints, great wisdom or honesty.

G. *Conch (Shankha):* Considered a blessing of Lord Śiva, the conch motif is highly auspicious in Indian culture, its presence signifying purity, longevity, health and prosperity. Those who carry this symbol on their palm gain much respect. The symbol of the conch shell also denotes one destined to awaken people from their slumbering and complacency, uniting all to a common cause.

H. *Stars (Nakshatras):* The number of converging lines that form a star makes them either lucky or unlucky. Overall symmetry is another factor in proclaiming Nakshatras to be beneficial or otherwise. Star rays of regular length composed of three lines, that is, six-pointed, are deemed optimal. Crosses/four-pointed stars (of equal length) also prove beneficial, although less so than their six-pointed cousins. Both six and four varieties create opportunities and lucky breaks. Their junctures are said to act like crossroads, facilitating change. When seen directly on planetary mounds or bracelets, six-pointed stars give beneficial results. Stars positioned directly on the houses of Rāhu or Ketu herald danger or accident, regardless of point number or symmetry. Stars comprising more than six points are largely associated with misfortune or delays.

I. *Water Pot (Jala Kumbha):* Signifies ancestral wisdom, its presence upon (or near) any Primary Line indicating contribution to ancestral wisdom and accrued experience. Like fish, the orientation of a Water Pot is highly important. An upturned pot signals lost or spilled energy; when righted, its contents are preserved. Orientation of pots also indicates their chosen application. If righted, one benefits throughout life; and all lines feeding into this pot are passed forward, benefiting a future incarnation. Upturned pots indicate that their contents are being inappropriately wasted for personal gain. Water Pots are most frequently seen on or near the house of Ketu.

J. *Spear (Shūla):* This symbol means to pierce or wound, and is considered to adorn the palms of warriors. In modern times this might equate to those in military service, police, game hunters, fighters or athletes. It might also apply to those who revel in open-conflict or highly competitive environments. Spears also signal swiftness and directness, their presence denoting those able to take decisive action in the face of confusion or adversity. Spears were symbolically thought to give one courage and/or the will to conquer.

K. *Bow*[30] *and Arrow (Śara Chāpa):* An auspicious symbol often said to adorn the palms of kings and princes. The presence of a bow and arrow indicates honour, strength and directness of character. When both are seen in unison, an individual attains fame and honour while seeking to serve the greater good. Solitary bows indicate those who also gain notoriety, but who serve only their inner desires.

L. *Eight-Pointed Discus (Asta Chakra):* This symbol is formed by two interlocking squares; its presence signifies satisfaction and attainment of many worldly desires. The eight-pointed discus aids in securing many fixed assets, but also incurs expenses in the upkeep and ownership of such assets. Those displaying this mark often feel trapped by wealth, acquiring many ancillary burdens and worries connected to their finances.

M. *Umbrella/Parasol (Cḥatra):* Considered a potent status symbol in Hinduism, Jainism and Buddhism, shading the heads of kings, honoured leaders or senior clan members. The presence of this symbol on the palm denotes those destined to assume some position of authority, such as a trusted minister, kingly advisor or judge. Umbrellas/parasols on either hand may indicate ancestral connections to former positions of authority.

N. *Drum (Damaru):* The dual-headed drum is an occult symbol, used by alchemists to symbolise the unity of opposition. Drums are often symbolic of deeper undercurrents that move beyond normal perception, likened to the pulse of life itself. The presence of a Damaru on the palm is thought to be an insignia of Shaivism, its bicameral structure echoing the interplay between masculine (Śiva) and feminine (Shakti) energies. See 'A. Crescent Moon (Chandra)' for similarities of interpretation.

O. *Mace (Gāda):* Similar to *Shūla*, though not to be confused. Gāda represents warriors of superior physical strength, those who punish wrongdoers or champion the weak. The mace, as a symbol of power, indicates a will to triumph against overwhelming odds; it also denotes honour upon the battlefield or *gāda-yuddha* (one skilled in war and weaponry).

P. *Plough (Hala):* Considered both weapon and agricultural tool, a plough upon the palm was thought to tie the fortunes of that individual to the land. The presence of Hala also denoted those most likely to unearth 'buried treasures' or those who prosper by their own handiwork. Hala were generally considered an auspicious symbol, however their presence may denote austerity, simple pleasures or a headstrong character.

FINGERPRINTS (HASTĀ-MUDRĀ)

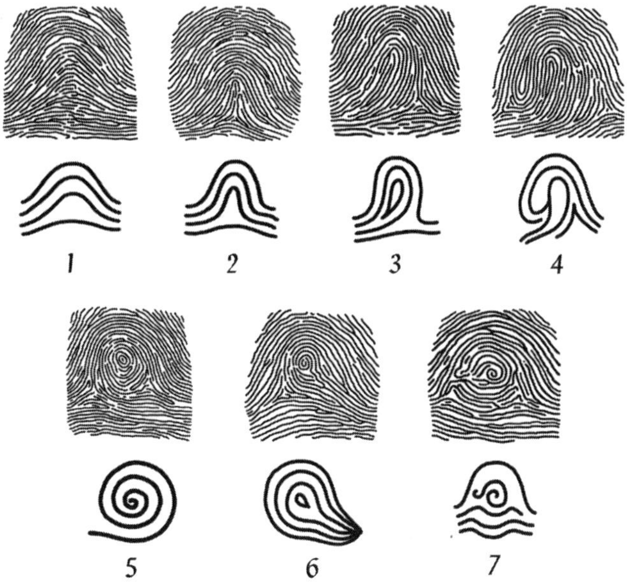

Modern fingerprint categories include: (1) arch, (2) tented arch, (3) loop, (4) double loop, (5) whorl, (6) pocked loop and (7) mixed.

Study and interpretation of the subtle depressions at the tips of fingers is known as *dactyloscopy*.[31] Today dactylograms (or fingerprints) help fortify forensic sciences in their detection (and prevention) of crime. Conveniently, modern appraisals group fingerprints into four basic patterns: arches, loops, whorls or mixed. Fine-tuning these patterns introduces three subcategories, namely: tented arch, double loop and pocked loop. Amongst the general populace, loops appear more prevalent, followed by whorls and, lastly, arches.

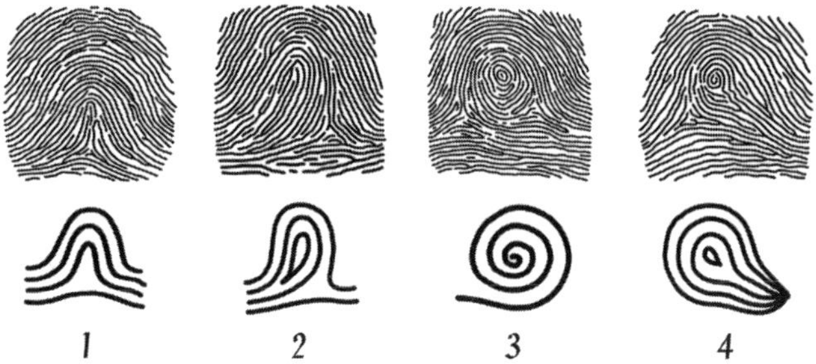

(1) Pitcher/Kalasha, (2) Conch/Shanku, (3) Disc/Chakra (open) and (4) Peacock Feather/Myurpiccha (closed).

Vedic palmistry generally considers three variations of fingerprint: Pitcher, Conch and Disc, the last sometimes differentiated into open or closed discs likened to the eye on a peacock's tail feather. A rough correlation of categories (traditional and modern) might be: Pitcher = arches and tented arches, Conch = loops and double loops, Discs = whorls and pocked loops. The remaining mixed categories, as their name implies, carry structural components of more than one type and so are generally defined by their dominant structures.

Like a human iris, fingerprints are unique to their owner – no two individuals display identical patterning. While fingerprints remain unchanged throughout life,[32] individual fingers may display more than one repeating print pattern; indeed, it is common for one or more fingers to show a variant pattern. This same variant will almost certainly be mirrored on the opposite hand. Variant patterns become important in Hastā Rekha analysis, specifically in regard to the finger upon which it is located and its corresponding planetary or shared planetary lord: for example, ring finger = Sun and Mars.

By modern standards, traditional divisions may seem simplistic; but numerically the number three is of great import to the Vedic sciences: for example, Sattva-Rajas-Tamas, Vāta-Pitta-Kapha, Brahmā-Śiva-Vishnu. The divisions and iconography of fingerprints do seem to be strongly founded upon the energetics of *Trimūrti*, Hinduism's sacred triad of gods: Brahmā (the creator), Vishnu (the preserver) and Śiva (the destroyer). Interpretations for mudrā/prints are given in Table 4.1.

Table 4.1 Interpretations for mudrā/prints

Pitcher/ Kalasha	**Brahmā**	Ranging from mild undulations to sharply rising tented peaks, pitchers make for grounded, practical and respectful thinkers, enjoying a detailed plan, strategy and creative solution. This fingerprint inspires confidence and loyalty, yet seldom adapts quickly to a fast-changing environment. Drawn to the arts and other creative endeavours, it indicates precision, coordination and balance
Conch/ Shanku	**Śiva**	Introverted and cautious, this mudrā is known for its supportive and friendly demeanour. Seldom taking risks, it prefers non-turbulent, peaceful environments, feeling comfortable to just go with the flow. Conch may turn inward (toward the little finger) or outward (toward the thumbs), its orientation mirrored on the opposite hand

Discs/ Chakra	**Vishnu**	Ranging from near circular to ovoid, Discs are independent, driven and of a cutting-edge temperament, with a gift for inspiring and enthusing. Regarded as aloof, calculating or cold, they are hardworking, analytical and quick-thinking, bringing urgency to any project (even if quickly losing interest themselves). The more compact the ridges of this structure, the greater their intensity
Peacock Feather/ Myurpiccha		This subgroup of discs are fiery in temperament with a flair for the dramatic. This structure is competitive, expressive and slightly unpredictable – drawn to demanding projects that require a high degree of creative thinking. The looser the ridges of this structure, the more unpredictable and aloof the character

TIMELINES (KĀLAMĀNA REKHA)

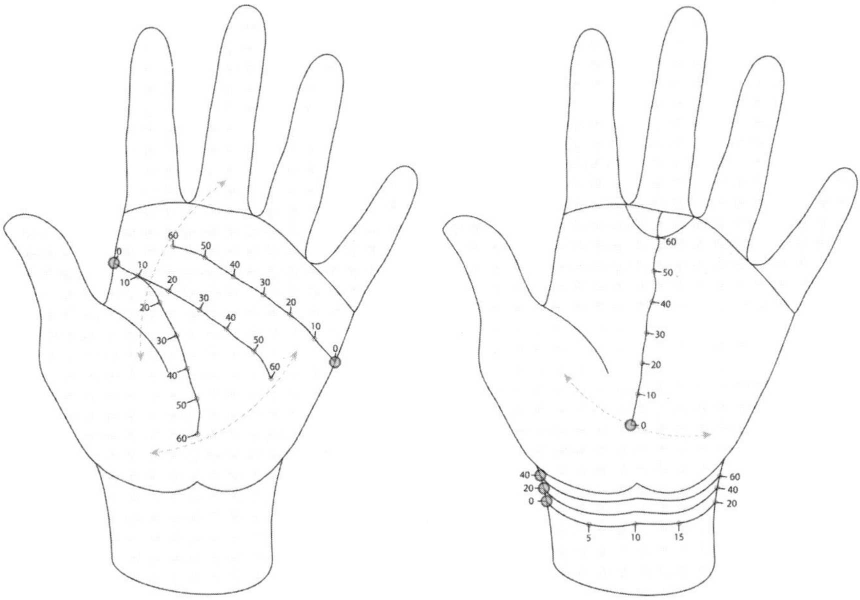

Timelines (Kālamāna Rekha) as measured on the palm. Left: Life, Head and Heart timelines. Right: Fate Line and bracelets. Note: Radial arrows denote average boundaries of Primary Lines as measured from year 0.

One powerful adjunct to the analysis of the lines are timelines. These are usually read from the four Primary Lines: Life, Head, Heart and Fate Lines,[33] plus the bracelets. Increments along these important lines anticipate the timing of significant life-events. Timelines are generally calibrated in cycles of 60 years, stepped off at their point of origin (see 0 on Primary Lines) and sequentially upward in the case of bracelets: Wealth (0–20 years),

Knowledge (20–40 years) and Devotion (40–60 years). These divisions may be subdivided as required.

(*Note:* Numbers 60 and 6 (6 + 0 = 6) are important in Vedic palmistry, associated with Pañcāṅgulī Devi (see Appendix): that is, the sixth zodiacal sign *Virgo* hosts *Hastā*, the hand (see Chapter 7). Six is also associated with planet Mercury (the healer) and ruler of the sixth zodiacal sign Virgo. Sixty and subsequently six are also the basis for an important Indian calendrical system known as Saṁvatsara,[34] based upon five Jupiter cycles equalling a period of 60 years.)

As a rule, most palms will show the Primary Lines somewhere in the region of the distances given in the diagram above; but of course not all will do so. For instance, the Life Line may extend right around the base of the thumb while others terminate well short of the example provided. Contrary to belief, short Life Lines do not herald short lives, they just provide the scale to be worked with and adjusted accordingly to as a period of 60 years always equates to its length. Having reached the end of the line a 61st year would again be taken from the initial '0' start point. This does not mean replaying childhood, teens and adulthood – but mental impressions, health scenarios or life-changing events of those years may again manifest in some form. This is why we say that elderly folk sometimes experience a kind of 'second childhood'.

In the case of foreshortened lives, serious health conditions or mental imbalances, some harmful influence should be detected upon one or more of the Primary Lines (usually all three), but even here there are cases where none were observed – yet life was cut short without showing any obvious signs on the palm.

In cases such as these, it should be remembered that extraordinary examples are not the norm and, while perplexing, should not be cited as a reason to abandon the whole ideology. Palmistry, like any complex system, is predicated upon multiple layers of sophisticated interaction, each part dependent upon the whole.

As my teacher once said to me: 'Information here (pointing at his palm) is 100% accurate, it cannot be otherwise. That which interprets Rekha (pointing to his head) may be flawed. Some things we cannot see or know at that time – that is the law of karma.'

NOTES

1. Deep, grooved lines are seen to be more earthy (Kapha) faint Rekha, more airy (Vāta) and medium Rekha with a pinkish hue (Pitta).
2. Life Lines are primarily identified with an individual's unique allocation of prāna or life-force.
3. Pitru = father.
4. Also known as Jeewan or Gotra Rekha.
5. Matru = mother.
6. Sometimes known as Dhana Rekha.
7. Chinese palmistry associates the middle finger (called Li) with the fire element.
8. Known as Solomon's ring in the western tradition of palmistry.
9. Also known as Brihaspati Mudrika.
10. Also Shani Mudrika.
11. Sādhanā = to accomplish or achieve moksha (liberation).
12. Known also as Shatru Rekha – line of enemies.
13. The mound of Mars sits directly below the origination point of the Life Line, indicating that these events are likely to occur sooner rather than later.
14. The regular use of stimulants such as tobacco, alcohol, recreational drugs and spicy foods are even more likely to vitiate Pitta dosha when a Mars Line is present.
15. Anurekha = major support line.
16. Also known as Lalana Rekha.
17. Also known as Dragon Lines.
18. Maṇibandha and Life Lines have deep unseen ties; afflictions to either can compromise longevity.
19. If the house of Ketu is supported by strong lines, it will in turn feed and strengthen bracelets.
20. In connection with traversing the seas, a typical signification of the Moon.
21. Also known as Sarasvatī Line.
22. Jupiter rules the element æther and in so doing acquires some lordship over the thumb. This association with contentment, expansion (feeling full) makes sense.
23. Also known as gridding.
24. Also Āchadita.
25. Signs and symbols are subject to some variance; the illustrations provided show the common points of agreement regarding their appearance.
26. Moon is a highly gregarious planet.
27. One popular sect of Hinduism, which embraces Śiva (and asceticism) as the Supreme Being, and true pathway to enlightenment.
28. Also known as Kamala.
29. Swastika = protected or kept from harm's way.
30. Also known as Dhanu (an archway or bow).
31. Another scientific nomenclature for fingerprints is dermatoglyphs (dermis = skin and glyph = inscription).
32. Fingerprints can be modified by diseases of the skin, or by self-mutilation such as with acid or heat. Criminals will sometimes try to mask fingerprints by these methods but in most cases make recognition of their prints more likely – due to partially obliterated dactylograms.

33. Some differences of opinion exist in regard to a timeline associated with Karma Rekha. It seems consistent to utilise a timeline here, as the remaining Primaries use timelines.
34. Jupiter's yearly transition through each zodiacal sign (Brahaspatya-varsha) varies between 155 and 390 days+; its sidereal revolution through the zodiac takes just less than twelve years. Saṁvatsara is a 60-year Jovian cycle, that is, 5×12 sidereal revolutions. Therefore, the cycle of Saṁvatsara offers yet another means by which our palmist/astrologer shines a light upon an individual.

PART III

PLANETS AND ZODIAC SIGNS

Chapter 5

PALMISTRY AND ASTROLOGY

As previously mentioned, palmistry and astrology are inseparable, either discipline requiring its would-be students to access identical core-level information. That is to say, planets (Grahas[1]) and zodiacal signs (Rashis[2]) remain fundamental to any understanding of their collective/predictive capabilities. Similarities between palmistry and astrology do not end there: use of *Nakshatras* (lunar mansions) also migrates to palm and fingers, their significations reflexed to those outlined in the horoscope. Additionally, palmistry presents something akin to the predictive timing or planetary periods – Dashas, as they are known in Jyotish. These are calculated using *Kālamāna Rekha*, literally meaning 'time-measurement lines', traced along the Primary Lines and bracelets (see Chapter 4).

INTRODUCTION TO THE PLANETS

One of the best ways to familiarise yourself with astrological precepts is to imagine all nine planets[3] Sun, Moon, Mercury, Mars, Jupiter, Venus, Saturn and lunar nodes (known as Rāhu and Ketu) functioning within the framework of a royal court (albeit a celestial one). Bound by their unique codes of friendship and enmity, each planet goes about its allotted duties – all of which naturally bring them into accord or conflict with one another. Table 5.1 outlines their various relationships and roles within the royal court. This information later becomes key in identifying suitable fingers upon which to wear gems. For more information see Chapter 12.

Table 5.1 Friendships, enmities and neutrality[4]

Sun (King)	*Friendship:* Moon, Mars, Jupiter *Enmity:* Venus, Saturn *Neutral:* Mercury	**Mars (Commander-in-Chief)**	*Friendship:* Sun, Moon, Jupiter *Enmity:* Mercury *Neutral:* Venus, Saturn	**Saturn (Servants)**	*Friendship:* Mercury, Venus *Enmity:* Sun, Moon, Mars *Neutral:* Jupiter
Moon (Queen)	*Friendship:* Sun, Mercury *Enmity:* None *Neutral:* Mars, Jupiter, Venus, Saturn	**Jupiter (Advisor)**	*Friendship:* Sun, Moon, Mars *Enmity:* Mercury, Venus *Neutral:* Saturn	**Rāhu (Militia)**	*Friendship:* Jupiter, Venus, Saturn *Enmity:* Sun, Moon, Mars *Neutral:* Mercury
Mercury (Regent)	*Friendship:* Sun, Venus *Enmity:* Moon *Neutral:* Mars, Jupiter, Saturn	**Venus (Advisor)**	*Friendship:* Mercury, Saturn *Enmity:* Sun, Moon *Neutral:* Mars, Jupiter	**Ketu (Militia)**	*Friendship:* Mars, Venus, Saturn *Enmity:* Sun, Moon, *Neutral:* Mercury, Jupiter

PLANETARY PORTRAITS

The following portraits hopefully create a framework upon which the reader may start to commit the essential planetary qualities to memory. Pictured as individuals, enmeshed in day-to-day activities animates the planets, lifting them from two-dimensional objects on the palm to three-dimensional characters with colourful life-stories. Once friendships, preferences and social hierarchy have been committed to memory, the job of assessing their immediate states and strengths should begin to leap from the palm and their stories unfold.

(*Note:* There are literally unending correlations between planets, people, places and objects; in fact, anything and everything that impacts upon the senses is considered to be a signification of a particular planet. The following portraits represent a fraction of these correlations, and should in no way be taken as exhaustive.)

SUN (SÛRYA)

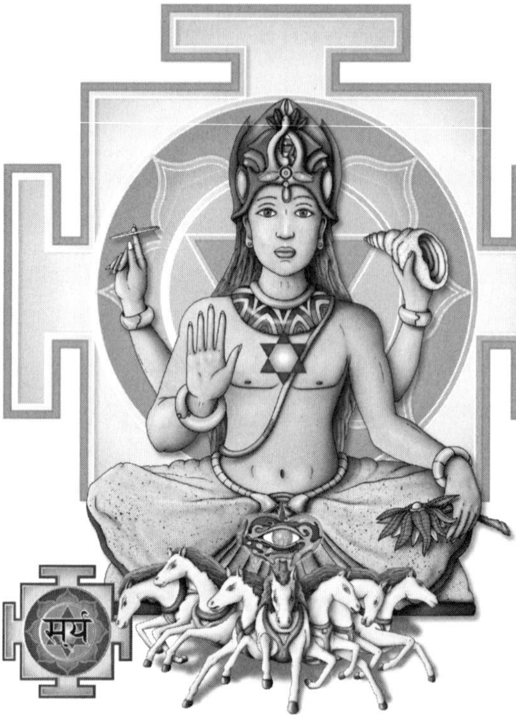

> The Sun, whose strength lies in a southerly direction, whose nature is like that of Raja (warrior), dresses in fine red silks and fire coloured ornaments, whose light and heat radiate outward. Representative of Atma, he rules Ayana (solstices). The chariot of the sun is pulled by seven horses (symbolising the seven spectral colours), his metal is swarna (gold).
>
> *Forty Vedic Hymns*

Dressing in fine red silks, Sûrya is considered the lord of planets (grahapati), his caste is warrior (Raja). Masculine in stature, with a blood red complexion, his element is fire, his guna Sattva (see Chapter 3). The light of Sûrya energises all planets (nodes excluded). Sun represents both Atma (true-self) as well as ego; he embodies unicity. His effects mature in the 22nd year of life. A decisive planet in career opportunities, Sûrya represents status and respect; he is happiest in southerly skies (at midday) or when associated with the fire Rashis (Aries, Leo or Sagittarius). Friendly toward Moon, Mars and Jupiter he shows enmity toward Venus and Saturn. Sûrya maintains cordial relations with Mercury. Sun is exalted in the sign Aries and rules Leo, his day is Sunday.

The Sun rules power; he can elevate an individual beyond all expectations and in some instances he can literally make one a king. Sûrya is representative of an individual's relationship toward figures of authority, be it father, business associates, corporations or financiers. More importantly, he dictates how those same authorities will react toward the individual. His persuasion method is punishment, his glance is upward, his shape is a circle. The colour of the sun is crimson, his taste is pungent (heating).

Sûrya holds dominion over the following:

General	Father, King, government, egotism, courage, self-respect, confidence, energy, vitality, ambition, nobility, generosity, truth, will-power, profession, status, solutions, ostentation, pomposity, despotism, idiosyncrasies and baldness
Natural World	Lions, tigers, ruddy goose, forests, strong and massive trees, rare woods, pine trees, cedar tree, deserts, gold, rubies and sunstone
Environments	Palaces, governmental buildings, temples/places of worship, magnificent buildings, large buildings, great halls, open areas, wooded areas and parks
Occupations	Economics, governmental, administration, physicians, royal appointments, pharmacies, chemical industry, drug manufacture, wool and mills, property surveying, jewellery, forestry management and photography
Health and Vitality	Heart, bones, eyesight (right eye), digestion, migraine, fevers, burns, cuts, dental problems, loss of appetite, cold extremities, neuralgia, poor blood circulation, diarrhoea and anaemia
Foods and Spices	Wheat, almonds, nutmeg, peppers, fine wines, rare liqueurs, spicy food, cayenne pepper, chilli peppers, black pepper, cinnamon, aromatic herbs
Hastā Rekha	Favourable Solar signs: well-developed Anamika (ring finger) or Sûrya-sthana, Keerthi or Punya Rekhas

MOON (CHANDRA)

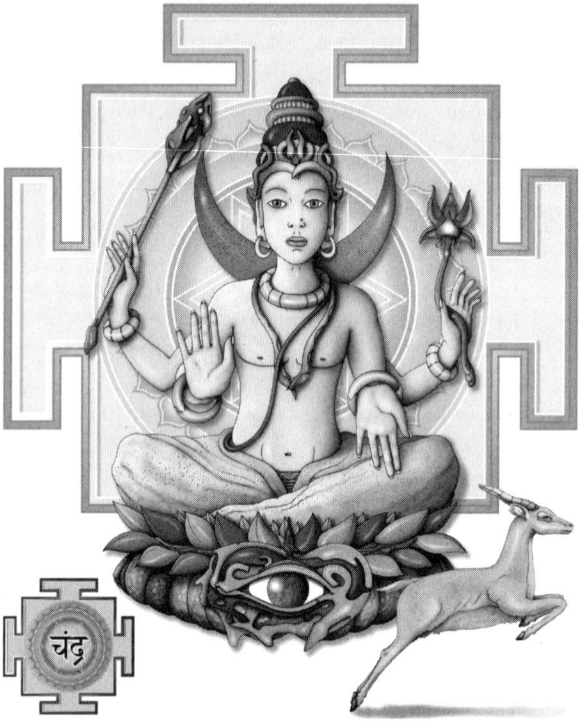

> Moon, whose strength lies in a northerly direction, whose nature is like that of a mother cow (kamadhenu); dresses in fine white silk and snow white ornaments, who exudes soma (nectar) that falls and spreads upon the earth, seeding all divine herbs. The chariot of the moon is crafted from rajata (silver) and pulled by ten white horses.
>
> *Forty Vedic Hymns*

Dressing in fine white silks, Moon is referred to as the queen of the night (Niśeśa), attaining maximum strength when full. Merchant (velanda) by caste and feminine in stature, Moon is tawny of complexion and Sattva in guna; her element is water. The light of the moon empowers all Nakshatras (lunar mansions). The Moon signifies mother and nurturing, that is, those that would keep us from bodily harm. Moon is typically seen as reflection of our true solar nature (see 'Sun (Sûrya)').

When strong, Moon exudes emotional maturity and clear thinking; if weakened or over-stimulated, she provokes self-obsession, over-sensitivity and depression. In matters of health, Moon presides over Rakta/blood, its quality and abundance (see 'Seven Tissues (Sapta Dhātu)' in Chapter 13), healthy lubrication of the tissues, complexion and vision. Moon rejuvenates and nourishes, helping to retain moisture and integrity through salts and secretions. Moon is always 'newly clothed' and short in stature, her method of persuasion is comfort, her glance is straight ahead. Moon is represented by a square, its colour is pale, its taste salty. Her effects mature in our 24th year of life. Moon is considered representative of chitta (consciousness), gaining strength in a northerly direction or when associated with the earth signs: Taurus, Virgo or Capricorn. Moon is exalted in the sign Taurus. Friendly toward Sun and Mercury, the Moon shows little enmity toward any planet, its Rashi is Cancer, its day Monday.

Chandra holds dominion over the following:

General	Mother, queen, women, beauty, romance, nurturing, home, security, comfort, emotional heart, softness, maternal instincts, reflective, romance, night-time, feelings, emotions, the body, growth, receptivity, fertility, aesthetic sensibilities, coolness, sailing, music, poetry
Natural World	Hare/rabbit, antelope, deer, vegetation, plant sap or oils, lotus flower, lily, jasmine, lily, slippery elm, comfrey, pearls, conch, moonstone
Environments	Seas, rivers, wells, springs, pools, aquariums, beaches, rivers, house-boats, welcoming places, comfortable hotels and guesthouses, healing sanctuaries
Occupations	Travel/tourism, welfare, agriculture, salt-mining, shipping, water sports, pearl farming, dairy/milk production, fishing, customs, mass media/general public, advertising, cafés/refreshments, healing centres, hospitals, manufacture of mirrors, plant nurseries and glass making
Health and Vitality	Stomach, lungs, breasts, eyes (left), blood, emotional heart, kidney/bladder, uterus, ovaries, loss of taste, mental disorders, depression, constipation, diabetes, anaemia, itching, dry skin, boils, coughing and swellings
Foods and Spices	Watery fruits (such as melon), coconut, root vegetables, cucumber, honey, cheese, milk, butter, ghee (clarified butter), rice, corn, stewed foods, all fermented foods
Hastā Rekha	Signs of excess lunar influence: well developed Chandra-sthana and/or Chandra Rekha may indicate self-obsession, depression or states of hypochondria

MERCURY (BUDHA)

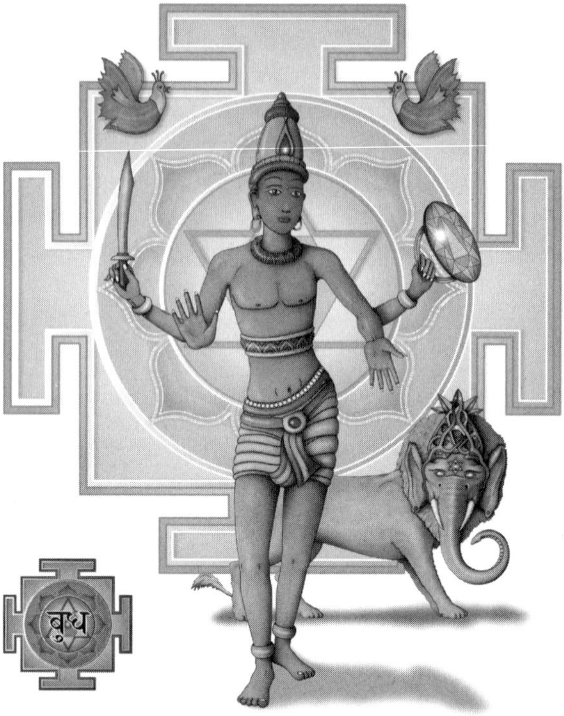

> Budha: who rules Mithuna (Gemini) and Kanya (Virgo) is green of body and ornaments. Seated upon a lion, his limbs encircle Mount Meru, his strength lies in an easterly direction. His symbol is an arrow, his metal is Pārada (quicksilver).
>
> *Forty Vedic Hymns*

Dressing in fine black silks, Mercury is youthful in appearance and mannerism. Fond of word-play and witticism, he is merchant by caste and Rajas in guna, his sex is neuter. Likened to the colour of grass, his taste is *shad-rasa* (six tastes[5]). Symbolically, Mercury is the planet of health and healing, specifically aiding in the lustre of the skin and the functionality of the lungs; his element is earth. Mercury matures in the 32nd year of life, his clothes are pristine (and fashionable), his stature is of average build, his movements are nimble and precise, his metal is quicksilver.

Master of buddhi (perception), he is analytical and curious by nature. Over-stimulated or tainted by strong external influences, his ability to remain neutral is quickly compromised. His method of persuasion is diplomacy, his glance sideways. Happiest residing in the east or associated with the air Rashis Gemini, Libra or Aquarius, Mercury is friendly toward Sun and Venus, but shows enmity toward Moon. To all other Grahas he maintains cordial relations. Mercury is exalted in his own sign Virgo and rules both Gemini and Virgo; his symbol is an arrow in flight, his day is Wednesday.

Budha holds dominion over the following:

General	Intelligence, dexterity, willingness, trading, mercantile pursuits, detachment, fascination, meticulousness, perception, charm, wittiness, comedy, entertainment, communication, daydreaming, contradiction, nervousness, astrology, magic, occult studies, childishness, naive, aloofness, fraudulent, double dealing, calculative, negotiator, entrepreneur, restlessness, movement and travel
Natural World	Lion, elephant, parrot, fruitless trees, bitter fruits, kusha grass (*Desmostachya bipinnata*), young green leaves, wild flowers, fresh herbs, sandalwood oil, mercury (Hg), emeralds, green peridot
Environments	Places of businesses, ports and airports, post offices, accounting departments, schools, playgrounds, places of non-violent sport, open parks, bookstalls, libraries, print shops, internet cafés, information/tourist centres
Occupations	Merchant/trader, accountant, writer, journalist, publishing, lawyer, public transport, crafts, travel agent, astrologer, stationer, teaching (educating), postman, translator, linguist, typist (office work), fraudster, mathematician, physician, physicist, gem-dealer, counsellor, advertising, bookseller
Health and Vitality	Skin (itchiness), lungs, hands and arms, colon and piles, nervous system and sensory disorders, brain diseases, insomnia, grinding of teeth, worry, palpitations, anxiety, impotency, vertigo and epilepsy
Foods and Spices	Mung beans, millet, mint, basil, chamomile, seedless fruits, GM crops, green vegetables, food additives, fast (convenience) foods
Hastā Rekha	Favourable signs of Mercury: Budha-sthana, Budha Rekha or well-developed Kanishtha (little finger), nimble/dexterous fingers, smooth skin

MARS (KUJA)

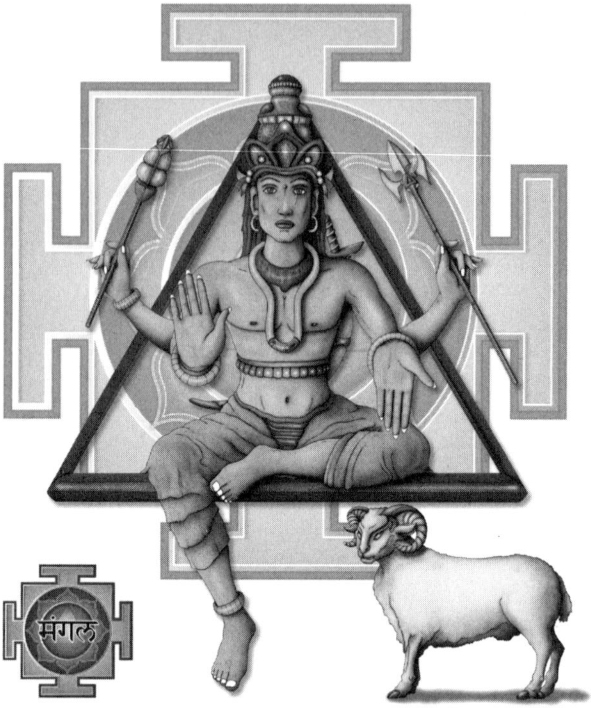

> Kuja; ruling Mesha (Aries) and Vrishchika (Scorpio), is red of body and ornaments. Powerful like Yamaraj, he is four limbed; his symbol is trikona (having three angles). Born of Bhūmi (Earth), he faces southward toward the infernal regions (and Yamaraj), his metal is loha (iron).
>
> *Forty Vedic Hymns*

Dressing in coarse red fabrics, Mars is short in stature with blood-red complexion, his persuasion method is punishment, his glance upward. Considered representative of power (shakti), his guna is Tamas. Mars is fierce and of a practical disposition, he promotes strong musculature, flexible sinew and a will to conquer. His movements are cutting and decisive. Symbolically, planet Mars represents courage, conflict and war, his metal is iron. Warrior by caste, he is masculine, his taste is pungent, his element fire, his symbol is a triangle.

Mars promotes strength (bala), aggression and survival instincts. He is happiest in a southerly direction (infernal regions) or associated with the earth signs Taurus, Virgo or Capricorn. Friendly toward Sun, Moon and Jupiter, he shows enmity toward Mercury but maintains cordial relationships with Venus and Saturn. He lords the signs Aries and Scorpio and is exalted in Capricorn, his day is Tuesday, his effects mature in the 28th year of life.

Kuja holds dominion over the following:

General	Soldiers, armies, commander-in-chief, fighters, physical prowess, dexterity and coordination, heroism, muscle, passion, goal-orientated, energy/shakti, aggression, sex, blood, surgery, injury, accidents, mechanical/technical ability, incisive thinking, strategy, alcohol, aphrodisiacs, buildings
Natural World	Ram, wolf, jackal, vulture, monkey, strong (flexible) woods, thorny trees, red flowers, red coral, red agate, carnelian, iron
Environments	Military bases, battlefields, military vehicles, munitions factory, chemical plants, abattoirs, butchers shops, shipyards, torture chambers, steel foundries, heavy construction, canteens, places of violent sports, hospital surgeries, A&E units
Occupations	Soldier, policeman, sports person, surgeons, younger siblings, building surveyor, engineers, metal polishers and gilders, chemists, military historians, builders, cooks
Health and Vitality	Maṃsa (muscle tissue) and majjā (bone marrow; see 'Seven Tissues (Sapta Dhātu)' in Chapter 13), fevers, liver complaints, cuts, burns, bruises, rashes, ulcers, carbuncles, surgery, lowered immunity, slow wound healing, malabsorption of minerals, bleeding haemorrhoids, atrophied muscle, acute complaints and stabbing pains
Foods and Spices	Meats, fried foods, heavily spiced foods, garlic, onions, red pepper, nettles, barley, coffee, spirits (alcohol), tobacco, hashish
Hastā Rekha	Formidable Martian signs: well-developed Kuja-sthana, prominent Maṇgal/Shatru Rekha

JUPITER (BRIHASPATI)

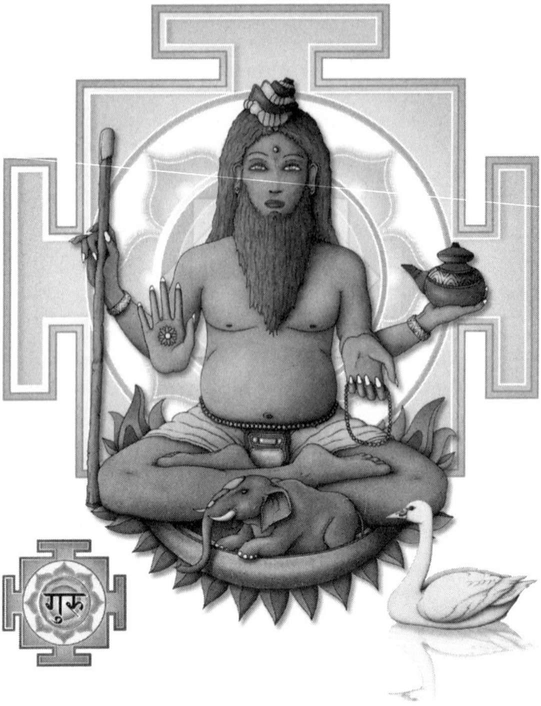

> Brihaspati: Ruling Dhanus (Sagittarius) and Meena (Pisces), his body and ornaments are of a yellow colouration. Four limbed, calm and mighty, he holds a rectangular water bowl. Facing in an easterly direction (toward the rising sun) his guna is Sattva, his metal is vanga (tin).
>
> *Forty Vedic Hymns*

Dressing in fine yellow fabrics, Jupiter is tall in stature with a complexion likened to saffron. Priestly (bamunu) by caste, his persuasion method is wise counsel, his glance direct. Considered the great benefic, Jupiter represents healthy discrimination, protection and devotion, his presence promotes Sattva, wealth, health and comfort. Indicative of healthy progeny, he enkindles knowledge, happiness and physical corpulence. Learned in shāstra (sciences and scriptures), he promotes philosophical insight and generosity. Jupiter is the significator for teachers, instructors and gurus. Masculine in sex, he is expansive and pervasive in demeanour, his taste is sweet, his element æther, his symbol a rectangle.

Happiest in an easterly direction (facing toward sunrise), he gains strength in the water signs Cancer, Scorpio or Pisces. Friendly toward

Sun, Moon and Mars, he shows enmity toward Mercury and Venus, yet maintains a cordial relationship with Saturn. He lords the signs Sagittarius and Pisces and is exalted in Cancer, his day is Thursday, his effects mature in the 16th year of life.

Brihaspati holds dominion over the following:

General	Gurus, teachers, leaders, advisors, counsellors, children, religion, philosophy, expansion and excesses, wealth, prosperity, fortunes, foreign aid, foreign investment, pilgrimages, friends, elder siblings, humanitarian acts, devotional nature, optimistic, lucky, genial, empathic, knowledge of shāstras, Hastā Rekha, Jyotish, Āyurveda, Vāstu, yogic studies
Natural World	Swan, elephant, goad, horses, sweet fruits, fruiting trees, ghee, milk, cream, sulphur, yellow sapphire, topaz, citrine
Environments	Schools, universities, libraries, law courts, bookshops, altars, shrines, monasteries, ashrams, banks, vaults, stock exchanges, fairs and festivals, charities, sacred rivers
Occupations	Teachers, spiritual instructors, ministers, bankers, financiers, IRS, treasurers, charity workers, lawyers, judges, auditors, editors, professors, scholars, sages, gurus, priests
Health and Vitality	Liver (enlarged), ears (hearing), medas (fat), allergies, excess Kapha, fatty tumours, lymphatic congestion, vertigo, water retention, flatulence, hernias, loss of memory, oedema, obesity
Foods and Spices	Ghee, butter, cream, milk, milk-rice, sugarcane, jaggery, rye, nuts (especially cashews and almonds), saffron, squash, sesame seeds, sesame oil, liquorice, spearmint, peppermint
Hastā Rekha	Favourable Jupitarian signs: well-developed Tarjani (forefinger), Guru Chandrika, Dīksha Rekha and Jupiter-sthana

VENUS (SHUKRA)

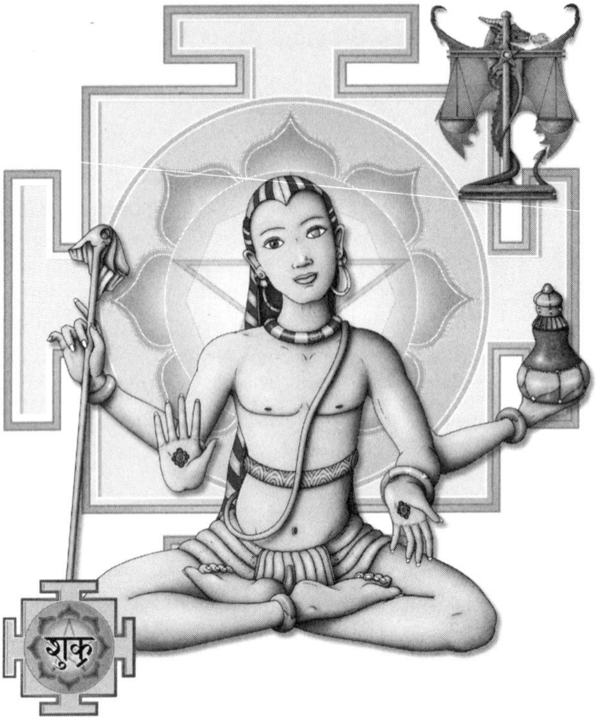

> Shukra: Facing northward, he is four limbed and peaceful. Seated upon a lotus flower bearing divine herbs, his symbol is a pentagram. White of body and ornament he is lord of Vrishabha (Taurus) and Tula (Libra), guru to all Asura, his metal is tamra (copper).
>
> *Forty Vedic Hymns*

Dressing in decorated (well-tailored) fabrics, Venus is of average stature with a variegated complexion. Priestly by caste, his persuasion method is coy glances and seduction. Considered a strong benefic, Venus is representative of physical potency (reproductive fluids), his presence enhances pleasure and creativity. Indicative of good looks, he is refined and learned in all scriptures (shāstras), his presence enkindles knowledge (for personal gain), happiness and physical indulgence. Venus hosts a disarming gentleness, appearing affectionate and defusing many potentially explosive situations. When strong, Venus indicates fullness of figure and smoothness of skin. Well versed in the musical arts, he is knowledgeable in all matters of the occult. Venus fortifies the immune system and supports our ability to procreate. Feminine in demeanour, his taste is sour, his element water.

Venus promotes luxury, his guna is Rajasic. Venus favours a northerly direction and the nighttime, he gains strength in the water signs Cancer, Scorpio or Pisces. Friendly toward Mercury and Saturn, he shows enmity toward Sun and Moon, yet maintains a cordial relationship with Mars and Jupiter. He lords the signs Taurus and Libra and is exalted in Pisces, his day is Friday. His effects mature in the 25th year of life, his symbol is a pentagram.

Shukra holds dominion over the following:

General	Spouse, lover, marriage partner, beauty, elegance, refinement, perfumes, romance, harmony, music, artistry, designer, fabrics, clothing, dance, flowers, courtier, minister, luxury, comforts, wealth, vehicles, vanity, proportion, sensual pleasures, laziness, magical arts, casting spells, palmistry and astrology
Natural World	Flowers, fragrant flowers, cotton, elephants, horses, polished woods, copper, diamonds, clear quartz
Environments	Film-sets, art galleries, car dealerships, clubs and nightclubs, casinos, music halls, theatres, high class restaurants, airport lounge, banquets, lavish hotels, ballrooms, beauty parlours, massage parlours, cinemas, brothels, opium dens, shopping malls, breweries
Occupations	Film stars, musician, artists, dancers, dramatists, jewellers, car dealers, fitness instructors, fashion designers, models, retail clothing, fabric manufacturers, make-up artists, fashion industry, shoe sales, hairdressers
Health and Vitality	Pelvis, menstruation, reproductive organs/genitalia, sexually transmitted diseases, kidney/bladder, eyes (iris), immunity, pancreas, liver and water metabolism, water retention (oedema), itchy skin conditions
Foods and Spices	Sugar, jaggery, dates, lotus seeds, oats, flour, sticky rice, cold foods, sweet drinks, liqueurs, cinnamon, cardamom, long pepper, saffron, desserts, all confectionery, icing
Hastā Rekha	Favourable Venusian signs: developed Shukra-sthana, Shukha mekhala and Sāntana Rekha

SATURN (SHANI)

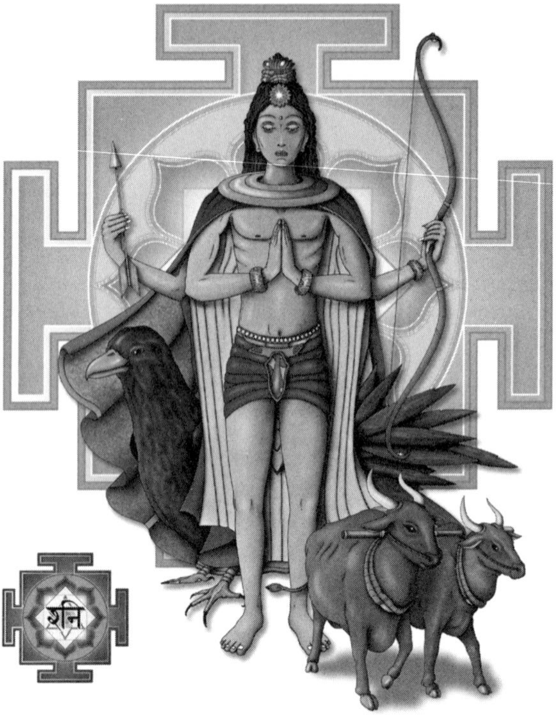

> Shani: is blue of body and ornaments, his direction is westward. His symbol is an archway, his eyes are blackened. Riding upon a crow, his caste is Śūdra (servant), his star is Bharani, his metal is nāgā (lead). Shani is lord of Makara (Capricorn) and Kumbha (Aquarius).
>
> *Forty Vedic Hymns*

Dressing in threadbare and aged fabrics, Shani is tall in stature with ashen complexion. Servant (Śūdra) by caste, his persuasion method is attrition, his glance frightful and downward. Considered a potent malefic, Saturn is representative of melancholia, rigidity and the withdrawal from worldly matters. Indicative of those who suffer under the yoke of tedious heavy work, his presence instils fear and depressive thoughts. Saturn relates to longevity, health and karma; when powerful he grants longevity, endurance and material gain (through hard work). Saturn is extremely people-unfriendly, preferring abstinence or solitude. Disciplined and resolute, he promotes liberation through suffering. Neuter in sex, his taste is astringent, his element is air.

Promoting dryness and decay, his guna is Tamas. Saturn is happiest in the westerly direction (facing sunset and the end of day), gaining strength in air signs Gemini, Libra or Aquarius. Friendly toward Mercury and Venus, he shows enmity toward Sun, Moon and Mars, yet maintains cordial relations with Jupiter. He lords the signs Capricorn and Aquarius and is exalted in Libra, his day is Saturday, his effects mature in the 36th year of life. Saturn's symbol is an archway.

Shani holds dominion over the following:

General	Longevity, asceticism, patience, delays, misery, depression, pain, suffering, loss of status, responsibility, sorrow, misery, fasting, famine, plague, poverty, decay, Tamas, loss of income, emaciation, putrid foods, crows, agriculture, root vegetables, old age, senility, constipation, injury through work, black magic
Natural World	Crows, buffalo, rats, locusts, weeds, root vegetables, parched earth, salt, rotten wood, heavily knotted woods, gnarled and twisted trees, lead, blue sapphires, blue amethyst
Environments	Hermitages, basements, subterranean caverns, wine cellars, mines, old people's homes, spiritual retreats, slums, sewers, refuse centres, junk yards, graveyards, abandoned houses, ruins, prisons and asylums
Occupations	Plumbers, all employees, servants, tenants, outcastes, eunuchs, elderly care, miners, gas fitters, iron and steel works, stonemasons, social services, orphanages, cheats and beggars, tinkers and scavengers, confidence tricksters, farmers and those who tend the land
Health and Vitality	Bone deformities, nerve damage, skin conditions, falling teeth, bowed legs and weak ankles, cancer, paralysis, epilepsy, all chronic illness, mental fatigue, asthma, rheumatism, arthritis, poor longevity, constipation, flatulence, bruises, blisters, loss of limbs, deafness, low immunity and infections
Foods and Spices	Black sesame seeds, maize, soybeans, peas, root vegetables, junk food, dried foods, putrid foods, foreign foods, vinegar, dry wine, triphala, myrrh, guggulu and frankincense
Hastā Rekha	Challenging Saturnine signs: developed Madhyama (middle finger), Shani-sthana, Shani Chandrika and Shani Rekha

LUNAR NODES (RĀHU AND KETU)

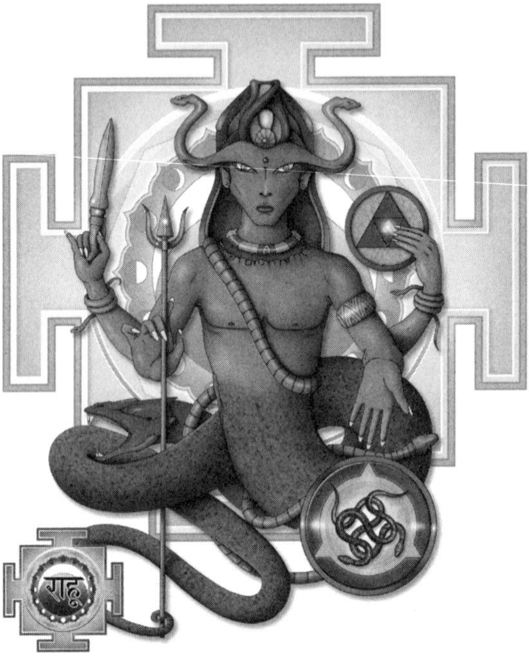

Rāhu – Northern node of the moon.

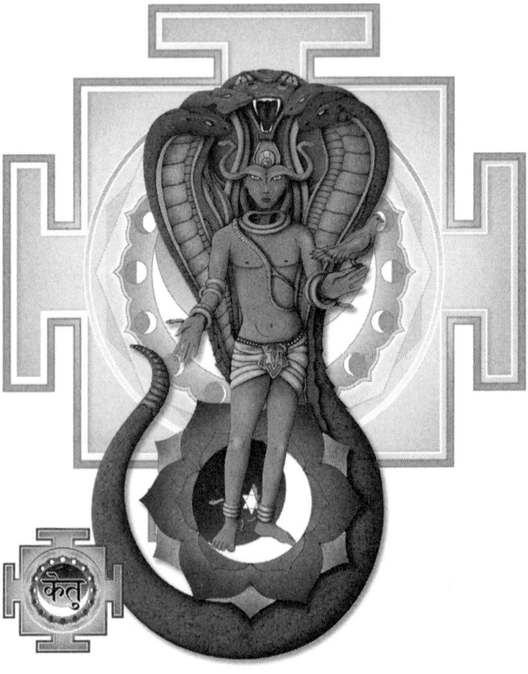

Ketu – Southern node of the moon.

> Rāhu: blue of body and of ornaments, his direction is south-westerly. Four limbed his teeth are fanged and irregular, his nature similar to that of the lion. His symbol is shoorpa (a winnowing basket), his metal pittala (brass). Ketu: variegated (multicoloured) of body and of ornaments, his direction is also south-westerly, his symbol a flag. Riding upon a lion his temperament is likened to Kuja, his presence associated with dhumaketu (comets) and smoke, his gaze is terrifying, his metal is kansya (bronze).
>
> *Forty Vedic Hymns*

Dressing in multicoloured robes, Rāhu is tall in stature and smokey-blue in complexion. Outcaste (mleccha),[6] his persuasion method is conspiratorial, his glance downward. Considered highly malefic, Rāhu rules insatiable appetites, psychotic episodes, dark desires, deranged thinking and a hunger for power. Rāhu revels in global communications and mass media, spreading confusion or frenzied rumours. Frequently this Graha is drawn to the darker 'addictive' aspects of life. Rāhu rules intoxicating substances, hallucinogens, toxic gases, poisons and chemicals. Neuter in demeanour, his taste is astringent, his element is air. Rāhu's symbol is a winnowing basket.

Rāhu promotes unrest and invention, his guna is Tamasic. Happiest in the south-westerly direction, he gains strength in the signs Virgo and Scorpio, prospering in all Rashis ruled by air (especially Gemini). Friendly toward Jupiter, Saturn and Venus, he shows enmity toward Sun, Moon and Mars, maintaining a cordial relationship with Mercury. Rāhu is without lordship of sign or day; however, likened to Saturn, he is given co-rulership of Aquarius and Saturdays. Rāhu's effects mature in the 48th year of life.

Rāhu holds dominion over the following:

General	Addictions, greed, power, māyā (illusion), deranged thinking, conspiratorial activities, snakes (particularly cobras), snake charmers, poisons, intoxicants, hallucinations, insect and reptile venom, astrology, foreigners, immigrants, a winnowing basket, ultraviolet (UV spectrum), mass psychosis, mass media, trends, insight, cutting-edge technology, fame, worldly desires, selfishness, illusionists, ghosts and ghouls
Natural World	Snake, raven/crow, jackal, wolf, scorpions, mosquito, anthill, owls, bug, any creature that has poison associated with its bite, dark forests, barren lands, brass, hessonite (also known as cinnamon stone)
Environments	Pharmaceutical labs, places with animals held in captivity, research facilities, nuclear power plants, toxic waste sites, slums, mines, oil refineries, mortuaries, graveyards, slaughter houses, electrical sub stations, mobile phone masts, wi-fi relays and routers

Occupations	Scientist, technician, research assistant, physicist or nuclear physicist, astronomers, pharmaceutical industry, magician, illusionist, entertainer (black comedy), any violent occupation, sex industry, manufacture of toxic medicine (petrochemical drugs), telephone engineer, aviation, computer programmer, mortician, slaughterhouse worker
Health and Vitality	Phobias, neurosis, psychosis, epilepsy, rheumatism, Vāta diseases, any incurable ailments marked by uncontrolled expansion or diversification (such as cancer), ulcers, skin diseases, tremors, indigestion, viruses, epidemics (contagious diseases), insomnia
Foods and Spices	Fast foods, microwave foods, colorants and additives, hydrated foods, preserved (dried) foods, calamus, sage, sandalwood, guggulu
Hastā Rekha	Challenging North Node signs: developed or darkened Rāhu Gṛha, Fate Line terminating near Rāhu Gṛha, Nakshatras (stars) on Rāhu Gṛha

Dressing in rags, Ketu is tall in stature, of a smokey-blue complexion and *varṇa-sankara* (of mixed caste). His persuasion method is violence, his glance downward. Considered highly malefic, Ketu is representative of mass catastrophes, psychic attacks and paranormal apparitions such as phantoms, ghosts and other disincarnate spirits. Ketu is significator for self-doubt, mass psychosis, fixations with the past, unconscious behaviour, nightmares, addictions and the participation in lost causes. He is frequently connected to poisons, poisonous people or toxic situations. Neuter in demeanour, his taste is pungent, his element is air.

Ketu promotes moksha (liberation and renunciation), yet his guna is Tamas. Happiest in the south-westerly direction, Ketu gains strength in the signs Virgo and Scorpio, prospering in all the fire signs (especially Sagittarius). Friendly toward Mars, Venus and Saturn, he shows enmity toward Sun and Moon, yet maintains a cordial relationship with Mercury and Jupiter. Ketu is without lordship of sign or day, but likened to Mars, he is given co-rulership of Aries and Tuesdays. The effects of Ketu mature in the 48th year of life, his symbol is a flag.

Ketu holds dominion over the following:

General	Global calamities, paranormal activity, apparitions, moksha (liberation), ascetics, enlightened beings, abstinence, unconventionality, un-diagnosable diseases, invisibility, compulsions, detachment, flags, historian, archaeologists, revolutions, occult powers, unsolved mysteries, other-worldly experiences, prisoners, murderers, lies, suicide, venomous speech, stuttering, foreign lands
Natural World	Savage dogs, snakes, biting animals, horned animals, bats, vultures, flying insects, burrowing creatures, maggots, bronze, chrysoberyl (cat's eye)

Environments	Graveyards, mountain tops, cyberspace, hidden monasteries, yogic retreats, sewers, burial grounds, crossroads, foul smelling/dirty places
Occupations	Undercover investigators/internal affairs, archaeologists, historians, forensics, taxidermy (skulls, hides and skins), mortician, bone mill and slaughter houses, refuse collection, sewage processing
Health and Vitality	Vāta type fevers, diseases which create a loss of structural integrity, malabsorption, diseases causing slow imperceptible damage, un-diagnosed sickness, epidemics, uncontrolled itching, boils, burning feet, slow-healing wounds, cancers, skin abbesses, bleeding disorders and spasms
Foods and Spices	Fast foods, spicy foods, food additives, red colorants, pickled or fermented foods, foreign foods, sage, calamus, juniper, ginger, gotu kola, skullcap
Hastā Rekha	Challenging South Node signs: developed or reddish Ketu Gṛha, Fate Line emanating from or Life Line terminating on Ketu Gṛha, Nakshatras (stars) on Ketu Gṛha

Chapter 6

PLANETARY MOUNDS AND ZODIACAL SIGNS

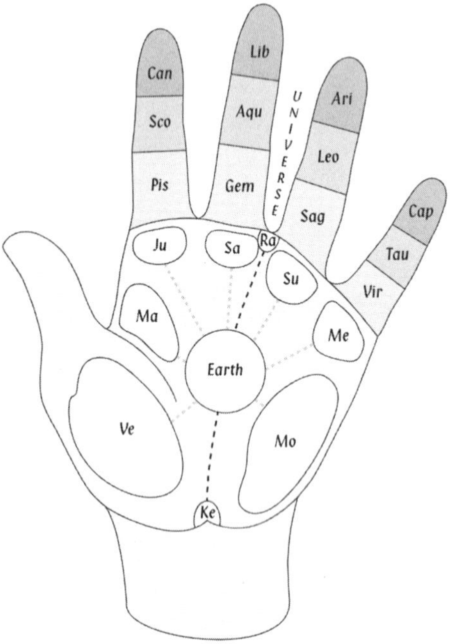

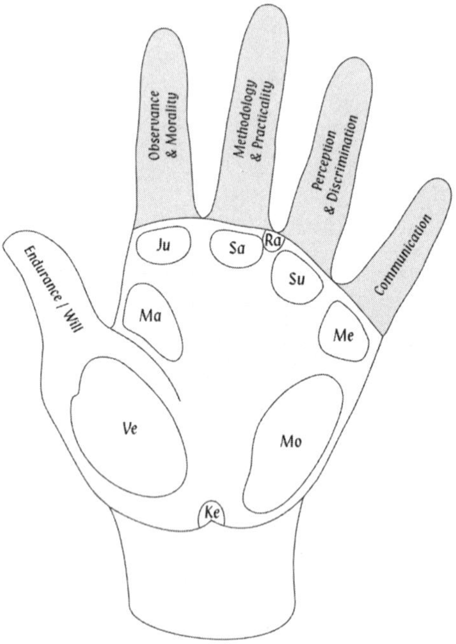

Left: Planetary mounds (parvata), lunar nodes (Rāhu and Ketu) and zodiacal signs (Rashis). Vedic Palmistry places the Earth at the centre of the palm, representing the plane of reference and the individual. Right: Qualities of the fingers and thumb, endurance and will (thumb), morality and observances (forefinger), practicality and methodology (middle finger), perception and discrimination (ring finger), communication and speech (little finger).

PLANETARY (PARVATA[7]) MOUNDS

Knowledge of planet and sign positions on the palm is critical to any appreciation of this discipline. Here, four planets are given direct rulership over the fingers (excluding thumb), leaving Moon, Venus and Mars to align themselves toward those fingers allocated as friendly[8] (see Table 5.1).

Compensation for these latter planets is to preside over substantially larger areas of palm. Lastly, Earth (resting centrally) represents the individual, the focal point for all planetary rays,[9] represented here by the central faint broken lines. Earth's location at the centre might also be thought of as the reference plane, reminding us that astrology is an Earth-centred science.

Parvata or planetary mounds are identified by the spongy pads situated at the base of each finger and at the sides of the lower palm. These mounds are allocated to Jupiter/Ju (forefinger), Saturn/Sa (middle finger), Sun/Su (ring finger) and Mercury/Me (little finger). Mars/Ma is identified by a raised 'triangular' plain lying just below the mound of Jupiter and above that mound allocated to Venus/Ve. The lunar mound, or Moon/Mo, is situated directly opposite that of Venus.

LUNAR NODES

Identification of those areas assigned to the lunar nodes can be a little more complex. Although awarded planetary status in astrology, Rāhu and Ketu are in reality shadows (chāyāgrahas). Similarly, their manifestation upon the palm remains veiled, revealed only by inference or lines. The home of Rāhu or *Rāhu Gṛha* often appears as a small depression or horizontal line, driving a wedge between the mounds of Sun and Saturn. The hand bearing more prominent signs of Rāhu indicates activities arising in this lifetime; the alternate hand, his influence or activity in a previous incarnation. The location of Ketu's home or *Ketu Gṛha* remains a slightly easier affair as its position is often marked by the symbol 'Λ' or that of an upturned water pot (see 'Symbols (Chinha)' in Chapter 4). Situated close the lower edge of the palm, Ketu's house is usually centred above bracelets – known also as Dragon Lines.[10]

In the illustration above, I have reproduced the figurative 'UNIVERSE' text – shown just above Rāhu's house. Its positioning here was explained to me as representing the unknown, a void between Saturn (karma) and Sun (Ātma[11]). This significant point of exit from the palm is bordered by the signs Gemini and Sagittarius, the latter defined astronomically as the sign closest to the galactic centre,[12] the former its anti-centre. The house of Ketu remains firmly anchored to the bracelets, an area associated with ancestral ties/blood lines and previous incarnations, as well as reflecting an individual's innate constitutional strengths and weaknesses.

ASTROLOGICAL SIGNS (RASHIS)

The twelve zodiacal signs have been allocated one phalange of the four fingers, grouped by element (see Chapter 2), air, fire, water and earth: that is, water (jala) signs relate to the index finger, air signs (vāyu) to the middle finger, fire signs (tejas) to the ring finger and earth signs (prithvi) to the little finger. Broadly speaking, the water element is representative of knowledge, or more specifically the retention of knowledge. The earth element relates to manifestation or material gain. The fire element relates to perception, assimilation and power – fire makes one 'like a warrior'. The air element relates to change, movement and relocation. Additionally, signs are arranged according to energetic, so Chara (dynamic and active signs) are furthest from the palm, ie. the tips of the finger. Sthira (fixed/resistant) are located at the middle phalange, held centrally, and Dwiswabhava (dual signs), having both qualities, are positioned at the base of the finger, closest to the palm.

A cursory glance at the allotment finger phalanges to zodiacal signs reveals that signs of exaltation (see Chapter 5) favour fingers ruled by the appropriate planet; so, for instance, Saturn, who prospers in air signs, finds his exaltation sign (Libra) appropriated to the tip of the middle finger, with the two remaining air signs Aquarius (own sign) and Gemini (friend) positioned comfortably above his planetary mound. Likewise Jupiter, prospering in water signs, finds his sign of exaltation (Cancer) appropriated at the tip of the forefinger, with the two remaining water signs Scorpio (friend) and Pisces (own sign) positioned comfortably above his planetary mound.

So, can a planetary placement of some significance (witnessed in the horoscope) be reflexed in some way on the appropriate finger phalange? This is an interesting question and one that requires more research. When I put this question to my tutor he seemed less positive, saying that in his opinion this technology had not been conveyed to the current generation of palmists; like other aspects of this work it seems to have fallen into decline. He did, however, note that a preponderance of *Sarala Rekhas* or simple lines, running vertically or horizontally on a particular phalange, seemed to highlight the importance of certain signs. Additionally, one variation of fingerprint (mudrā; see 'Fingerprints' in Chapter 4), on one of the four fingertips, also signalled some noteworthy relationship to one of the four moveable signs Aries, Cancer, Libra or Capricorn.

PORTRAITS OF RASHIS

Table 6.1 represents a general overview of the twelve signs and *some* of their more commonly agreed qualities.[13]

Table 6.1 The twelve zodiacal signs and some of their qualities

Rashis	Qualities
Sign: Aries (Mesha) **Ruler: Mars** **Symbol: Ram** **Element: Fire**	Masculine and of reddish complexion, its element is fire, its lord Mars. Mesha is warrior by caste, its guna Rajasic, its symbol a ram. Adventurous and risk-taking, the temperament of Aries is dynamic, excitable, decisive and easily irritated (they do not suffer fools gladly). Aries is prone to diseases of excess Pitta dosha, that is, blood toxicity, excess bile, enlargement of liver and itchy diseases of the skin. Mesha Jamna Rashi[14] often indicates a heroic, lustful or philanthropic character
Sign: Taurus (Vrishabha) **Ruler: Venus** **Symbol: Bull** **Element: Earth**	Feminine, sensual and pale of complexion, its element is earth, its lord Venus. Taurus is of merchant caste, its guna Rajasic, its symbol a bull. The Taurean temperament is methodical, tenacious and practical, having excellent stamina (physically and mentally). Taurus is prone to diseases involving vitiated Kapha dosha, that is, excess phlegm, respiratory weakness, swollen glands, heart conditions and stagnant lymph. Vrishabha Jamna Rashi indicates a forgiving, charitable and attractive character
Sign: Gemini (Mithuna) **Ruler: Mercury** **Symbol: Twins** **Element: Air**	Neuter of gender, with a grassy green hue, its element is air, its lord Mercury. Gemini's caste is servile, its guna Rajasic, its symbol twins holding a mace and lute (respectively). The Gemini temperament is erratic and animated, its mood changeable. Original in thinking, it is a highly adaptable and intellectual sign. Gemini is prone to diseases of excess Vāta Dosha creating dryness, aches, joint and muscle pains, moving (constantly relocating) pains, respiratory weakness including bronchitis or childhood asthma. Mithuna Jamna Rashi indicates a knowledge of scriptures, gambling and one who is pleasing to women folk
Sign: Cancer (Karkata) **Ruler: Moon** **Symbol: Crab** **Element: Water**	Feminine and of a pale red hue, its element is water, its lord the Moon. Cancer is priestly by caste, its guna Sattvic, its symbol a crab. The Cancer temperament is tenacious, reliable, communicative, thoughtful, hospitable, fair and intellectual. Cancer is prone to diseases of excess Kapha dosha such as bronchial/nasal congestion, abdominal bloating, nausea, digestive disorders (stomach-related) and ulcers. Karkata Jamna Rashi denotes individuals short in body, longer in limb, effeminate in disposition
Sign: Leo (Simha) **Ruler: Sun** **Symbol: Lion** **Element: Fire**	Masculine and of pale complexion, its element is fire, its lord the Sun. Leo is of warrior caste, its guna Sattvic, its symbol a lion. The Leo temperament is dynamic, ambitious and warm-hearted. Sometimes given to arrogance or excessive procrastination, it also inspires self-confidence and loyalty. Leo is prone to diseases of excess Pitta dosha such as: fevers, inflammation, heart disease, hypertension, rheumatic fever, weakness of vision. Simha Jamna Rashi indicates those of short tempers, proud, valiant and sure-footed
Sign: Virgo (Kanya) **Ruler: Mercury** **Symbol: Virgin** **Element: Earth**	Feminine and of fair complexion, its element is earth, its lord Mercury. Virgo is of merchant caste, its guna Tamasic, its symbol a youthful maiden. The Virgo temperament is shy, child-like, over-analytical and over-sensitive, with a meticulous sense of inner-order. Virgo is prone to diseases of excess Vāta dosha such as: nervous disorders, skin conditions, digestive complaints (constipation). Kanya Jamna Rashi indicates a pious, wise and tender disposition

Sign: Libra (Tula) **Ruler: Venus** **Symbol: Merchants Scales** **Element: Air**	Masculine and of dark (black) complexion, its element is air, its lord Venus. Libra is of servile caste, its guna Rajasic, its symbol the scales of a merchant. Drawn to relationships, the Libra temperament is artistic, musical, judgemental, idealistic, changeable, and in some cases violent. Libra is prone to suffer problems in the area of the lower back, kidneys, bladder, urinary tract, spine and skin, as well as pancreatic imbalances. Tula Jamna Rashi indicates learned, tall and rich individuals
Sign: Scorpio (Vrishchika) **Ruler: Mars** **Symbol: Scorpion** **Element: Water**	Feminine and of reddish-brown complexion, its element is water, its lord Mars. Scorpio is priestly by caste, its guna Tamasic, its symbol a scorpion. Reclusive and defensive, the Scorpio temperament is tenacious, single-minded and acrid. Unmatched in its ability to accrue enemies, its forepart is sharp, its body slender. Scorpio is prone to suffer ailments of the urino-genital organs such as renal calculi, bladder infections, fistula, haemorrhoids, cystitis and venereal disease. Vrishchika Jamna Rashi indicates a respectable individual, likely to receive wounds, or suffer from bouts of repeated poisoning
Sign: Sagittarius (Dhanus) **Ruler: Jupiter** **Symbol: Bow/ Archer** **Element: Fire**	Masculine and of pale complexion, its element is fire, its lord Jupiter. Sagittarius is priestly by caste, its guna is Sattvic, its form that of a centaur bearing a bow.[15] The Sagittarius temperament is fiery, free-spirited, honest, god-fearing, straightforward and diligent. Prone to diseases of excess Pitta dosha, Sagittarius may experience: poor circulation, blood poisoning (tetanus), arteriolosclerosis, gout, thrombosis, stroke, rheumatic fevers and varicose veins. Dhanus Jamna Rashi is said to indicate a poet, artist or one learned in multiple shāstras
Sign: Capricorn (Makara) **Ruler: Saturn** **Symbol: Crocodile** **Element: Earth**	Feminine and variegated of colour, its element is earth, its lord Saturn. Capricorn is merchant by caste, its guna is Tamasic, its form is that of a quadruped (crocodile) bearing the tail of a fish. The Capricorn temperament is self-reliant, motivated and intellectual, it has an acumen for economics and politics. Capricorn may be prone to diseases of excess Vāta dosha such as: constipation, arthritis, paralysis, rheumatism, dental decay, sciatica, osteoporosis and abdominal distension. Makara Jamna Rashi indicates those prone to wonder or as having attractive eyes
Sign: Aquarius (Kumbha) **Ruler: Saturn** **Symbol: Water Bearer** **Element: Air**	Masculine, its element is air, its ruler Saturn. Aquarius is servile by caste, its guna is Tamasic, its form is that of a male figure cradling a pitcher of water. Future-orientated and progressive, the Aquarius temperament is idealistic, loyal, rational and inventive, preferring the unconventional viewpoint. Kumbha is prone to diseases of the circulatory system such as arterial hardening, numb extremities, water retention, itchy skin and impeded recovery from infection or wounds. Kumbha Jamna Rashi indicates those prone to steal from others or those wishing to share in the limelight of another
Sign: Pisces (Meena) **Ruler: Jupiter** **Symbol: Fishes** **Element: Water**	Feminine, its element is water, its ruler Jupiter. Pisces is priestly by caste, its guna is Sattvic, its form is that of a two-headed fish sharing a single tail.[16] Reserved and orthodox, the Pisces temperament is amenable, artistic and musical. Kind-natured and receptive, they are also indecisive or suffering from an inner malaise. Pisces may be prone to diseases of excess Kapha dosha such as: catarrh, congestion, excess stomach mucosa (nausea), high cholesterol, lipoma, oedema, gout, chilblains and itchiness. Meena Jamna Rashi indicates those who seek comfort, are religious and delight in travel

NOTES

1. A Sanskrit word meaning to seize of grasp.
2. A Sanskrit word meaning qualities ascribed to an astrological sign.
3. The trans-Saturnians (Uranus, Neptune and recently demoted Pluto) remained unknown to the ancients; however, the addition of the two luminaries (Sun and Moon) and lunar nodes (Rāhu and Ketu) brings the complement to nine.
4. As per *Brihat Parasara Hora Shāstra.*
5. All six tastes are important for the balance of health and dosha, these being: sweet, sour, salty, pungent, bitter and astringent.
6. Typically representative of non-Aryans, barbarians or Greeks. The science of astrology was known to be well established (and honoured) among the latter; hence Rāhu Graha became strongly affiliated with astrology.
7. Parvata = mountain.
8. The Moon, Venus and Mars have no finger allocated to them; see Table 5.1 to determine friendships and enmity between planets.
9. The powerful rays of the Sun are in turn retuned by each planet co-mingling their own energetics, such as colour, frequency, temperature, temperaments and so on. Planets' rays carry the specific energetics of each planet.
10. Maṇibandha (bracelets) are thought to be heavily influenced by the lunar nodes, hence their alternate name 'Dragon Lines'. Bracelets from bottom to top relate to wealth, knowledge and devotion.
11. Representative of soul.
12. For more information on the significance of the galactic centre see the author's previous work, *Jyotish: The Art of Vedic Astrology* (Mason 2017).
13. Qualities of Jamna Rashi from *Nārada Purāṇa.*
14. Also known as Chandra Lagna, that is, the sign occupied by the natal moon.
15. Alternatively, Shara Chāpa (bow and arrow).
16. Alternatively, tethered fish, swimming in opposite directions.

PART IV

NAKSHATRAS (LUNAR MANSIONS)

Chapter 7

NAKSHATRAS AND THE PALM

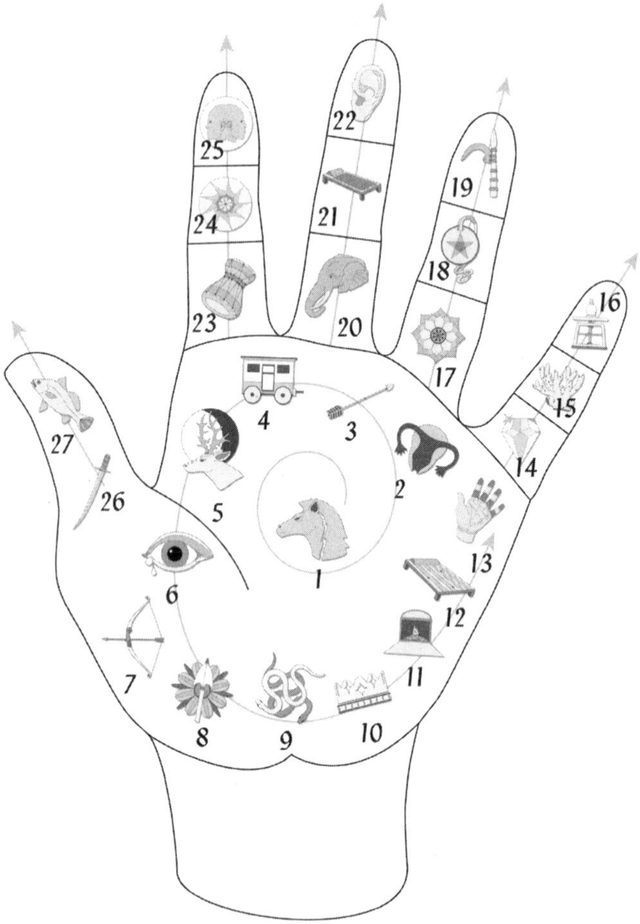

Nakshatras: (1) Ashwini, (2) Bharani, (3) Krittika, (4) Rohini, (5) Mrgashirsha, (6) Ardra, (7) Punarvasu, (8) Pushya, (9) Aslesha, (10), Magha, (11) Purvaphalguni, (12) Uttaraphalguni, (13) Hastā, (14) Chitrā, (15) Swati, (16) Vishaka, (17) Anuradha, (18) Jyestha, (19) Mula, (20) Purvashadha, (21) Uttarashadha, (22) Śravana, (23) Dhanistha, (24) Shatabhishak, (25) Purvabhadra, (26) Uttarabhadra and (27) Revati. Note: Positions are mirrored on both hands.

In this section we consider *Nakshatras*, sometimes referred to as Lunar Mansions. Nakshatras[1] form an integral and ancient part of the Vedic Astrological canon, their symbolism and usage appearing uniquely Indian. Although comparative astrological traditions such as Arabic *Manāzils* and the Chinese *Sieu* echo lunar divisions of space, their interpretation and usage appear to have lapsed over the ensuing centuries.

The word *Nakshatra* appears to have no definitive meaning, yet might be interpreted as 'those that protect' or 'endure', honouring some awareness of their antiquity and dependability in astrological analysis.

The significance of Nakshatras and their occupation by Moon, ascendant or planet is essential for any deeper understanding of a horoscope. The natal position of the Moon (in this regard) is especially important, due to its dominion over Nakshatras; indeed, one of the ancient names for Moon was *Nakshatra-nâtha* meaning 'Nakshatra lord'.

(*Note:* For the purposes of this section Nakshatras will refer to the Lunar Mansions (or divisions of space), whereas Nakshatra-Rekha will refer to star symbols found on a palm. The latter are identified as converging lines (three being optimal) and appearing anywhere on the hand. These latter Nakshatra-Rekha appearing on Graha-sthana, formed by lines of equal length and six points, are particularly auspicious. If Nakshatra-Rekha points exceed six, or their lengths remain unequal, they are to be considered more troublesome, said to represent obstacles or challenges. For more information see 'Symbols (Chinha)' in Chapter 4.)

Due to their distribution over the palm and fingers, there is no way to determine which planet (in that person's horoscope) tenants a particular Nakshatra – using only the hand. However, the presence of prominent star patterns (Nakshatra-Rekha) may reveal prominent Nakshatras, that is, those most likely to impact the individual's life. Similarly, symbols (see 'Symbols (Chinha)' in Chapter 4) that reside within the boundaries[2] of a particular Nakshatra are considered to work through the latter's influence (for more information see Chapter 10). Additionally, the presence of scars, moles or inherited creases (these being caused by age or repetitive actions) may also activate the particular Nakshatra within which they reside.

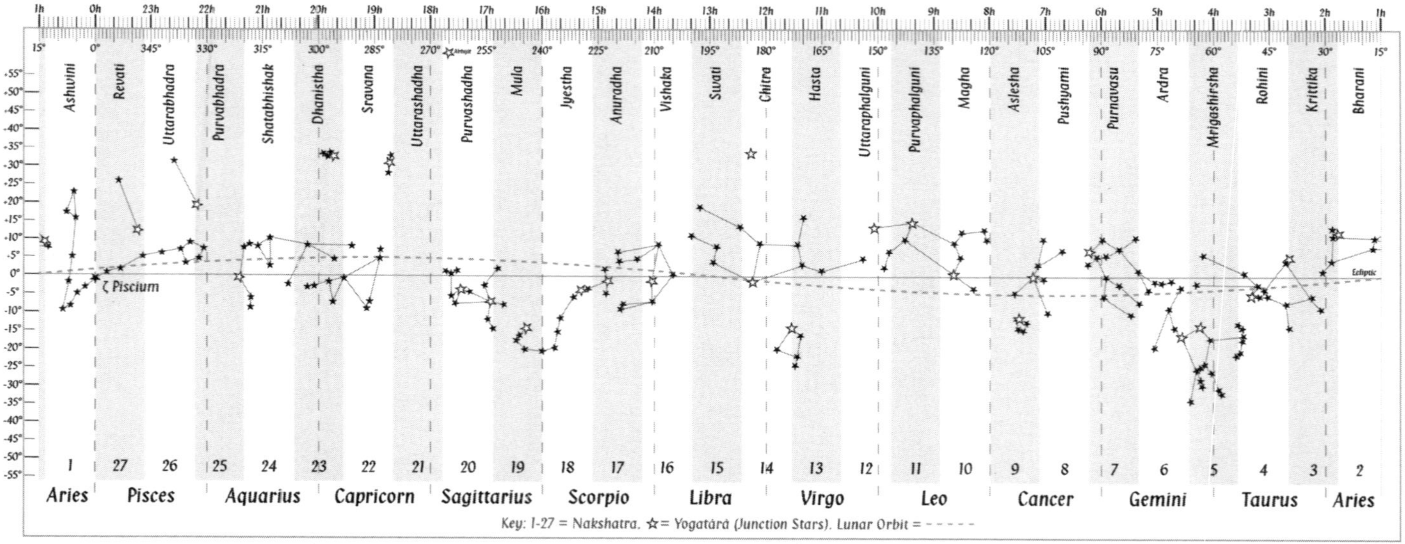

Nakshatra divisions superimposed over the zodiac. Revati Yogatârâ (ζ Piscium) represents the datum point (0° Aries). Large white stars = Yogatârâ or junction stars, central straight line = ecliptic, and broken undulating line = confines of the lunar orbit.

Chapter 8

NAKSHATRAS AND JYOTISH

At this point its probably worth giving a brief account of Nakshatras and their esteemed position in Hastā Rekha and Jyotish.

Each Nakshatra represents a 1/27th division of the sky,[3] or to put it another way, the progression of the Moon in any given 24-hour period (albeit an idealised increment[4]). The alternating grey-white horizontal bands in the image show these idealised increments. Over the course of 27 days and 7+ hours the Moon completes a sidereal (fixed star to fixed star) orbit. The word *sidereal* means 'pertaining to stars'.

The astr-ology and astr-onomy of ancient India appears to have initially favoured lunar observation. This in part may stem from the swift and convenient motion of the Moon across our skies as well as its accommodating level of illumination, which allows stellar observations to be made at any point along its orbit. Having both star and Moon visible = efficient sky mapping. Over a 24-hour period the Moon travels somewhere between 12° and 15° along (or at least close to) the ecliptic.[5] As astrology is principally centred upon stars and zodiac, individual increments of Nakshatras were calculated by dividing the ecliptic (360°) by 27, equalling a unit of 13° 20'. Within each division, a prominent star called a Yogatârâ was elected to represent its portion or boundary. Identification of these Yogatârâ enable an observer to make a quick assessment of the Moon's monthly progress. However, from a cursory glance at the Nakshatra divisions diagram it is quickly noted that Yogatârâ are not equidistant and in some instances stray dramatically from the lunar orbit.[6] It therefore becomes apparent that Nakshatra divisions are idealised 'mathematical' boundaries only. This fact is reinforced by the ancients themselves, who aptly referred to the zodiac as Manomaya Chakra or 'wheel of the mind'.

In Vedic Palmistry, this lunar cycle is similarly migrated to the hand, its motion or evolution of Nakshatras no longer an undulating heavenly path, but instead becoming a spiralling motion, moving outward from the palm's centre up through the mounds of Sun, Saturn, Jupiter and Mars and down over the thumb, following the contour of the lower palm, over the mound of

Venus and then Moon. As the spiral again rises along the palm's percussion, it crosses Mercury's mound before ascending each of the fingers in the sequence – from little finger to ring finger, to middle finger to forefinger, before finally ascending the thumb.

Chapter 9

LUNAR MYTHOLOGY

Mythologically, the Moon (called Chandra) may be either masculine or feminine, according to his/her situation. With regard to Nakshatras, the Moon takes on a masculine role, as husband to these 27 lunar brides. During his monthly cycle he might be said to 'rest' in the arms of each bride for a single day and night.

Generally care free and of a happy disposition, it is said Chandra started to became infatuated with his fourth bride, Rohini.[7] Wishing no longer to leave her side, he eventually became stationary. Naturally, his remaining 26 wives quickly became vexed and decided to punish him. To teach him a lesson they placed a consumptive curse upon their husband. Sitting back, they waited for his orb to shrink and his light to fade.[8] As the Moon's body grew slimmer, the nights grew darker, nourishment[9] of the crops ceased as vegetation upon the earth began to wither and die.

Before the world perished, Chandra's curse was lifted by Lord Śiva, who, believing the Moon had learnt his lesson, felt the time had come to reinstate the luminary to his former glory. By his adherence to a number of powerful rasāyana drugs,[10] administered by Śiva himself, the Moon again grew strong, bright and full; however, despite this excellent recovery, Moon continues to suffer his old affliction, re-experiencing consumption each month – lest his desires for Rohini return. As a consequence of this action, Moon is continually reminded to attend to the needs of all wives.

And what of Rohini?

She continues to steal a few extra minutes from Chandra during each monthly interlude, a phenomenon borne out astronomically as well as astrologically as the unique orbit of the Moon does indeed appear to prolong his transit through Rohini Nakshatra – at certain latitudes.

Chapter 10

NAKSHATRA QUALITIES AND THEIR PROPITIATION

The following is a reproduction of an early attempt to organise and categorise Nakshatras. Taken from the sixth century AD *Brihat Saṃhitā* (*Functions and Properties of Asterisms*), Nakshatras are divided into seven groups, each expressed in terms of fixed, sharp, fierce, swift, tender, sharp/tender and mutable. Here we gain some inkling into Nakshatra usage well over a thousand years ago.

Each of the seven categories have been assigned their preferred activities – that is to say, those undertakings best suited to a lunar transit through their allotted degrees (Table 10.1). For example, Ashwini, Pushyami and Hastā Nakshatras are considered swift, favourable for medical treatment, trading, study and generally pursuing pleasurable activities. Likewise, during palm analysis, the qualities of Nakshatras influence those Rekha or chinha found tenanting their allotted positions.

Table 10.1 Nakshatra functions and properties

Fixed *Nakshatras*	Sowing seeds or planting trees, royal coronations, financial investments, propitiation acts and the laying of foundation stones
	Rohini, Uttaraphalguni, Uttarashadha, Uttarabhadra
Sharp *Nakshatras*	Mantra, spells and incantations, raising of spirits, seeking alliance with kings, dispensation of law and the incarceration of wrong-doers
	Ardra, Aslesha, Jyestha, Mula
Fierce *Nakshatras*	Capture of wrong-doers, defeat of enemies, working with poisons, lighting fires, forging, manufacture of weapons
	Bharani, Magha, Purvaphalguni, Purvashadha, Purvabhadra
Swift *Nakshatras*	Medical treatment, healing, short journeys, trading, pleasurable pursuits, artistic endeavours, study/education, buying or wearing fine clothes and the adornment of gemstones
	Ashwini, Pushyami, Hastā

Tender *Nakshatras*	Propitiation of gods, wearing fine clothes, adornment of gemstones, artistic endeavours, performance of music, forming friendships or sexual union
	Mrgashirsha, Chitrā, Anuradha, Revati
Sharp/Tender *Nakshatras*	Propitiation of gods, devotional acts (see also Sharp and Tender rows)
	Krittika, Vishaka
Mutable *Nakshatras*	Communication, education, study, long and short pilgrimages, devotion to one's chosen deity and the offering of ghee, honey and scented flowers
	Punarvasu, Swati, Śravana, Dhanistha, Shatabhishak

Just as planets and signs are placated (or strengthened) via remedial measures (see Chapter 12), similarly Nakshatras are propitiated to obtain or relieve their effects.

Table 10.2 represents a slightly more modern guide to Nakshatra usage as here a composite has been assembled from a number of astrological texts, including *Brihat Saṃhitā, Nakshatra Chudamani* and Purāṇic sources,[11] as well as material from currently practising astrologers in Śrī Laṇkā and India.[12]

Table 10.2 Modern guide to Nakshatra usage (sample table)

Sinhala	Sinhalese equivalent
Tārā/Stars	Fixed star designation (astronomy)
Rashi/Sign	Corresponding astrological sign
Chinha/Symbol	Popular symbol used to identify Nakshatras
Gaṇa/Temperament	Nakshatras are categorised as divine, human or demonic
Jāta/Sex	Masculine or feminine
Ruling Planet	Planetary overseer
Dosha	Vāta, Pitta or Kapha
Shakti	Predominant energetic expressed
Maha Guna	Sattva, Rajas or Tamas
Varna/Caste	Brahmin, warrior, merchant, servant, farmer, butcher or outcaste
Chāndramāsa/Lunar Month	Synodal month (full moon to full moon)
Karma/action and Kāraka/significations	Karma = appropriate action/s undertaken under the auspices of that Nakshatra. Significations = actions/objects most likely to be influenced by that Nakshatra
Devata/Deity	Primary presiding deity
Pooja/ceremonial items	Appropriate items to honour that Nakshatra
Ahuti/Fire ritual	Fire ceremony, preferred offering and appropriate mantra
Nakshatrayoga	Remuneration for offerings made under the relevant Nakshatra

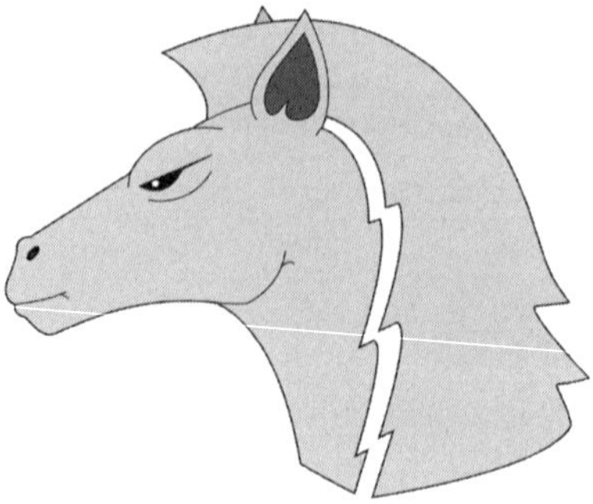

1. Ashwini

Sinhala	Ashvidha
Tārā/Stars	β and γ Arietis
Rashi/Sign	0° – 13° 20' Aries
Chinha/Symbol	Horse's head
Gaṇa/Temperament	Divine
Jāta/Sex	Masculine
Ruling Planet	Ketu
Dosha	Vāta
Shakti	Healing
Maha Guna	Rajas
Varna/Caste	Merchant
Chāndramāsa/Lunar Month	Āshvina (first half)
Karma/action and Kāraka/significations	Preparation of medicine, use of healing mantra, practice of astrology, construction of yantra, worship of guru/teacher. Travel, moving home, conveyances: including four-legged animals such as horses and elephants
Devata/Deity	Ashwini Kumaras: horse-headed twins, acknowledged for their healing skills and rejuvenative arts
Pooja/ceremonial items	Gold, black cloth, black gram, black sesame seed paste, Garuda (eagle), Kuchala,[13] lotus flower, white flowers, Sudha (calcium carbonate), sandalwood[14] or guggulu[15] incense, milk or milk-rice pudding.
Ahuti/Fire ritual	Milk-rice pudding, cast into fire 108 times with Gāyatrī mantra
Nakshatrayoga	Those offering horses, chariots/carriages under this star incur a future noble birth

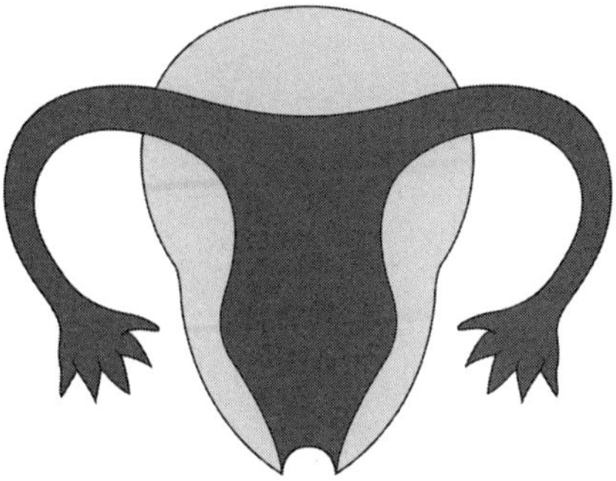

2. Bharani

Sinhala	Benara
Tārā/Stars	35, 39, 41 Arietis
Rashi/Sign	13° 20' – 26° 40' Aries
Chinha/Symbol	Yoni (female genitalia)
Gaṇa/Temperament	Human
Jāta/Sex	Female
Ruling Planet	Venus
Dosha	Pitta
Shakti	Bearing away
Maha Guna	Tamas
Varna/Caste	Outcaste
Chāndramāsa/Lunar Month	Āshvina (second half)
Karma/action and Kāraka/significations	Purification of sacred space with fire, removal of negative forces, construction of puṭa (burning pits), calcination of metals and minerals, drying of herbs, purgation of toxins, surgery, imprisonment, accidents, war (killing), gambling, theft, winning women and adventures
Devata/Deity	Yamarāj: lord of death and the underworld, he and his sister (Yami) become the first humans to ascend to Devaloka (godly realm)
Pooja/ceremonial items	Blue cloth, blue lotus, Amalaki,[16] Kāka (crow), Guggulu, Aguru[17] incense and jaggery rice
Ahuti/Fire ritual	Honey and ghee, cast into fire 108 times with Gāyatrī mantra
Nakshatrayoga	Those offering land or cattle to Brahmins under this star receive large numbers of cattle in a future birth

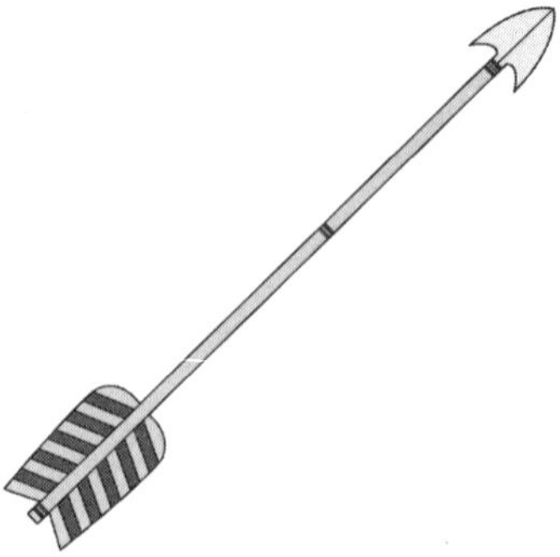

3. Krittika

Sinhala	Kathi
Tārā/Stars	η, 27, 23, 20, 19 and 17 Tauri
Rashi/Sign	26° 40' Aries – 10° 00' Taurus
Chinha/Symbol	Arrow in flight, sword, razor or edged weapon
Gaṇa/Temperament	Demon
Jāta/Sex	Feminine
Ruling Planet	Sun
Dosha	Kapha
Shakti	Cutting
Maha Guna	Sattva
Varna/Caste	Brahmin
Chāndramāsa/Lunar Month	Kārtika (first half)
Karma/action and Kāraka/significations	All fire rituals, worship of Lord Śiva, forging, sharpening metal, heating, burning, cutting, tearing, purifying, preparation of remedies that improve speech and intelligence, gaining siddhis through sādhanā[18]
Devata/Deity	Agni: fire god. A pivotal figure in Vedic literature, firstly co-creationist of the universe, later adopting the role of celestial messenger
Pooja/ceremonial items	Fig tree, Myura (peacock), honey, ghee, all red flowers but especially Karaveera,[19] ghee and guggulu incense
Ahuti/Fire ritual	Yoghurt and cooked rice, cast into fire 108 times with Gāyatrī mantra
Nakshatrayoga	Milk-rice prepared for the satisfaction of Brahmin under this star, attain merit in a future birth

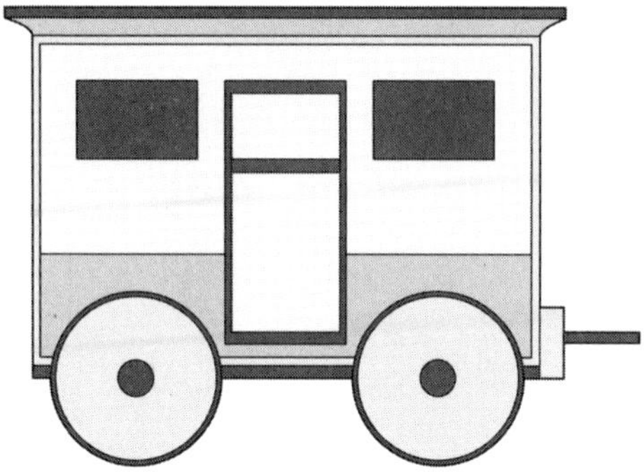

4. Rohini

Sinhala	Rehena
Tārā/Stars	α, θ1, θ2, γ, δ and ε Tauri
Rashi/Sign	10° 00' – 23° 20' Taurus
Chinha/Symbol	Cart, chariot or banyan tree
Gaṇa/Temperament	Human
Jāta/Sex	Masculine
Ruling Planet	Moon
Dosha	Kapha
Shakti	Growing
Maha Guna	Rajas
Varna/Caste	Śūdra
Chāndramāsa/Lunar Month	Kārtika (second half)
Karma/action and Kāraka/significations	Planting herbs and spices, purveying of wholesome foods, manufacture of perfumes, extraction of essential oils, construction, laying foundation stones, Vāstu (arrangement of sacred space), buying new homes, marriage, vehicles and the promotion of leadership
Devata/Deity	Prajapati: an epithet of Brahmā, frequently described as lord of all living creatures. Brahmā is first of three supreme divinities in Hinduism (collectively known as Trimūrti).
Pooja/ceremonial items	Sugarcane, Jambu,[20] lunar symbol, Hamsa (swan/goose), Sarasvatī, black cloth and flowers, black sesame seed paste, Brahmā statue, Tamala leaf,[21] Salai Guggulu,[22] milk rice, Kasturi[23] gland
Ahuti/Fire ritual	Mustard seeds and ghee, cast into fire 108 times with Gāyatrī mantra
Nakshatrayoga	Milk-rice prepared with ghee and served to Brahmins ends all indebtedness to ones ancestors

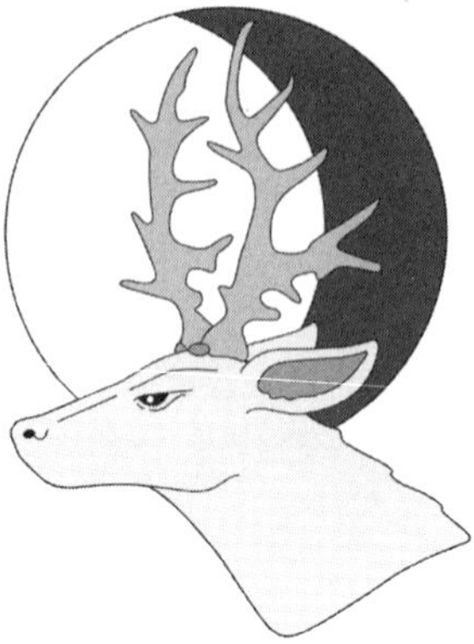

5. Mrgashirsha

Sinhala	Muwasirasa
Tārā/Stars	λ, φ1, φ2 Orionis
Rashi/Sign	23° 20' Taurus – 6° 40' Gemini
Chinha/Symbol	Head of a deer
Gaṇa/Temperament	Divine
Jāta/Sex	Feminine
Ruling Planet	Mars
Dosha	Pitta
Shakti	Searching
Maha Guna	Tamas
Varna/Caste	Farmer
Chāndramāsa/Lunar Month	Mrgashirsha (first half)
Karma/action and Kāraka/significations	Manufacture of rejuvenating medicine, rasāyana therapy, making ghee, collecting milk, honey, dates and almonds, yogic practice, bathing under moonlight, sādhanā, charitable acts, promoting a business
Devata/Deity	Soma: presiding over amrita (nectar), this deity takes on a number of guises in the Vedas, named and honoured, yet less anthropomorphic than his contemporaries. Soma later becomes synonymous with the Moon god – Chandra
Pooja/ceremonial items	Gold, white cloth, white flowers, lotus, Khadira,[24] Kukkuti (hen), Shadanga-dupa (six aromatic herbs, gums and resins), milk rice
Ahuti/Fire ritual	Milk rice and ghee, cast into fire 108 times with Gāyatrī mantra
Nakshatrayoga	One attains heaven if dairy cattle are offered on this day of this star

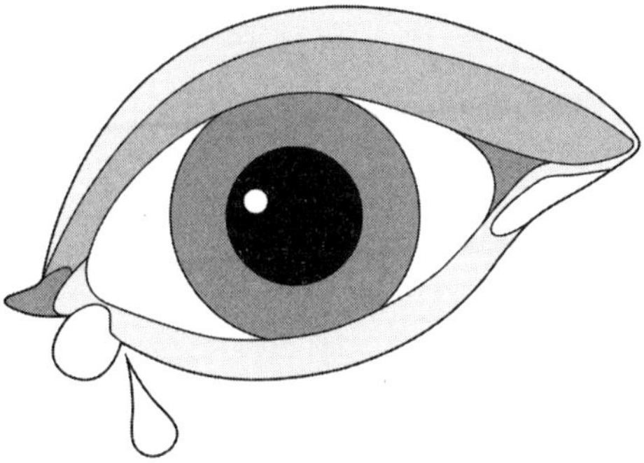

6. Ardra

Sinhala	Ada
Tārā/Stars	α Orionis and 134/135 Tauri
Rashi/Sign	6° 40' – 20° 00' Gemini
Chinha/Symbol	Teardrop
Gaṇa/Temperament	Human
Jāta/Sex	Feminine
Ruling Planet	Rāhu
Dosha	Vāta
Shakti	Moistening
Maha Guna	Sattva
Varna/Caste	Butcher
Chāndramāsa/Lunar Month	Mrgashirsha (second half)
Karma/action and Kāraka/significations	Purification and detoxification (purgation of visha/poison), defeat of enemies, exorcism of spirits, witnessing terrible things (trauma, struggles, torture, violence, accidents involving fire, etc.), worship of Rudra, overcoming the fear of death, feeding white cows
Devata/Deity	Rudra: an early Vedic storm deity, presiding over rain, cattle and health. Rudra later becomes synonymous with a wrathful incarnation of Śiva. Śiva is third of three supreme divinities in Hinduism (collectively known as Trimūrti)
Pooja/ceremonial items	White flowers, white sandalwood paste, Dattura,[25] white sesame seed paste, Khadira, Krouncha (heron), sesame paste, shali (red rice) Aguru
Ahuti/Fire ritual	Honey and ghee, cast into fire 108 times with Gāyatrī mantra
Nakshatrayoga	Offerings of sesame seed oil, ghee or abstinence from food on the day of this star ensure safe passage on perilous journeys

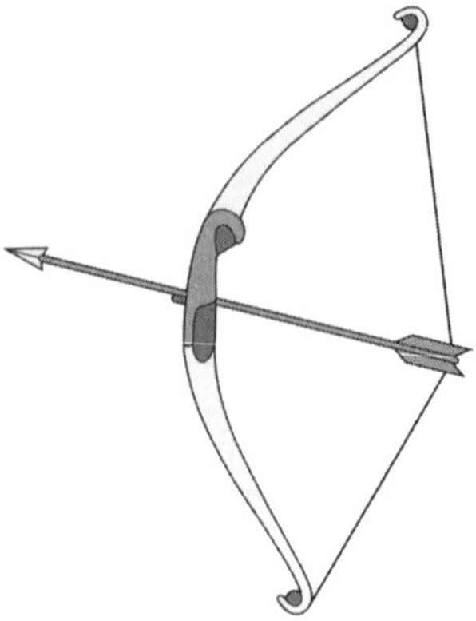

7. Punarvasu

Sinhala	Punawasa
Tārā/Stars	β and α Gemini
Rashi/Sign	20° 00' Gemini – 3° 20' Cancer
Chinha/Symbol	Bow or quiver of arrows
Gaṇa/Temperament	Divine
Jāta/Sex	Feminine
Ruling Planet	Jupiter
Dosha	Vāta
Shakti	Renewal
Maha Guna	Rajas
Varna/Caste	Merchant
Chāndramāsa/Lunar Month	Pushya (first half)
Karma/action and Kāraka/significations	Fasting, dietary changes, intake of foods rich in minerals, harvesting fruits, Āyurvedic study, taking medicines, Jyotish, Seemantham (ritual undertaken by pregnant women in odd-term months), educational rituals, new vehicles or travel
Devata/Deity	Āditi: mother to the twelve Ādityas, her name means 'boundless' or 'infinity'
Pooja/ceremonial items	Black cloth, bamboo, Hamsa (swan), mantra, boiled milk, saffron, white sandalwood paste, jasmine and jaggery
Ahuti/Fire ritual	Sesame rice and ghee, cast into fire 108 times with Gāyatrī mantra
Nakshatrayoga	Those offering bread on the day of this star are awarded birth into a wealthy family

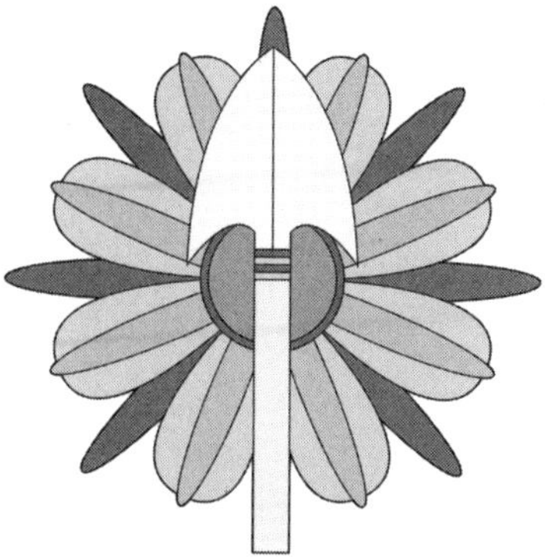

8. Pushyami

Sinhala	Pusha
Tārā/Stars	δ, γ, θ Cancri
Rashi/Sign	3° 20' – 16° 40' Cancer
Chinha/Symbol	Arrow head, flower or cow's udder
Gaṇa/Temperament	Divine
Jāta/Sex	Masculine
Ruling Planet	Saturn
Dosha	Pitta
Shakti	Nourishing
Maha Guna	Tamas
Varna/Caste	Warrior
Chāndramāsa/Lunar Month	Pushya (second half)
Karma/action and Kāraka/significations	Study of Vedas (scriptures), teaching, mantra, Jyotish, Āyurveda, worshipping of astra (weapons), removal of curses, pooja and attainment of siddhis
Devata/Deity	Brihaspati: instructor to the gods and Vedic warrior (armed with an iron axe). Later Brihaspati becomes identified with the planet god Jupiter
Pooja/ceremonial items	White cloth and flowers, Aswatha,[26] Jala Murgābī (waterhen[27]), yellow cloth, saffron and sandalwood, lotus flowers, burning Khadira wood (*Acacia catechu*) and rice yoghurt
Ahuti/Fire ritual	Milk and ghee, cast into fire 108 times with Gāyatrī mantra
Nakshatrayoga	Gold, given on the day of this star ensures the pleasure of all planets

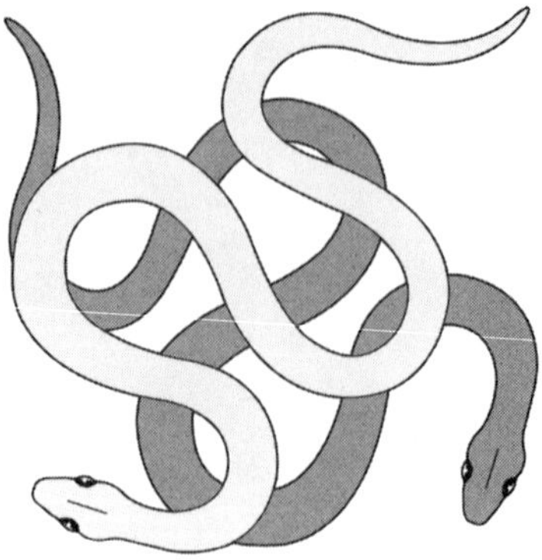

9. Aslesha

Sinhala	Aslisa
Tārā/Stars	ε, δ, σ, η, ρ and ζ Hydrae
Rashi/Sign	16° 40' – 30° 00' Cancer
Chinha/Symbol	Serpent
Gaṇa/Temperament	Demon
Jāta/Sex	Masculine
Ruling Planet	Mercury
Dosha	Kapha
Shakti	Entwiner
Maha Guna	Sattva
Varna/Caste	Outcaste
Chāndramāsa/Lunar Month	Mágha (first half)
Karma/action and Kāraka/significations	Practice or study of Jyotish, mantra against black magic, treatment of infection, removal of poisons, treatment of paralysis or viral illness, Ratnachikitsa (especially emerald), preparation of Maṇi bhasma, medicinal Visha (healing poisons), blaming, depression and suicide
Devata/Deity	Sarpa: one of eleven Rudras (Ekādaśarudras), Sarpa was the offspring of Tvashtar, artificer to the gods
Pooja/ceremonial items	Nagakeshara,[28] Tittibha (red-wattled lapwing bird), honey, red cloth (red-brown like the fur of a monkey), Haridra[29] root, brown/red flowers, a serpent idol, sandalwood paste, rice pudding and sweetened milk
Ahuti/Fire ritual	Ghee and Guggulu, cast into fire 108 times with Gāyatrī mantra
Nakshatrayoga	Silver attained on this day makes one fearless

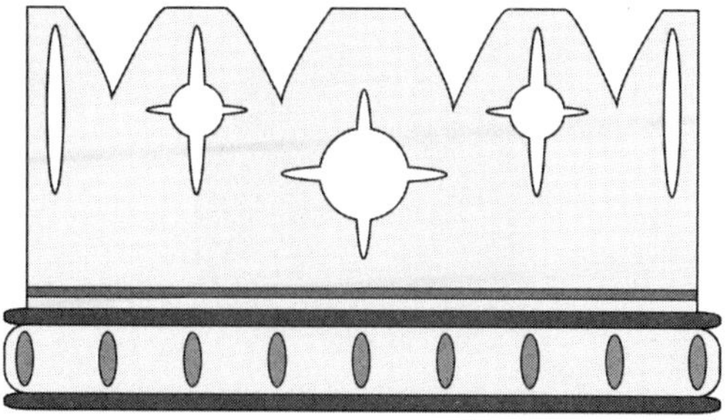

10. Magha

Sinhala	Maa
Tārā/Stars	α, η, γ1, ζ, μ, ε and ο Leonis
Rashi/Sign	0° – 13° 20' Leo
Chinha/Symbol	Crown or throne
Gaṇa/Temperament	Demon
Jāta/Sex	Masculine
Ruling Planet	Ketu
Dosha	Kapha
Shakti	Magisterial or mighty
Maha Guna	Rajas
Varna/Caste	Śūdra
Chāndramāsa/Lunar Month	Mágha (second half)
Karma/action and Kāraka/significations	Consulting learned individuals, formulating strategies, gambling, taking risks, all decisive actions, Pitri Tarpana,[30] Kanyadhanam,[31] recitation of snake bite mantra, digging wells
Devata/Deity	Pitris/Manes: progenitors/forefathers of mankind, warding over the fates of mankind
Pooja/ceremonial items	Vata (*Ficus bengalensis*), Champak (*Magnolia champaca*), black cloth, Kāka (crow), golden Pitru statue, Aguru, ghee and Guggulu incense
Ahuti/Fire ritual	Ghee, wheat flour and jaggery cast into fire 108 times with Gāyatrī mantra
Nakshatrayoga	Alms given on the day of this star are rewarded with cattle

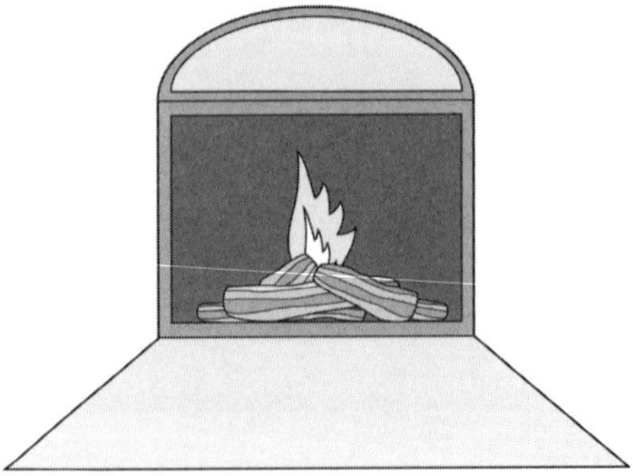

11. Purvaphalguni

Sinhala	Puwapal
Tārā/Stars	δ and θ Leonis
Rashi/Sign	13° 20' - 26° 40' Leo
Chinha/Symbol	Fireplace, cot or hammock
Gaṇa/Temperament	Human
Jāta/Sex	Feminine
Ruling Planet	Venus
Dosha	Pitta
Shakti	Enjoying, procreating
Maha Guna	Tamas
Varna/Caste	Brahmin
Chāndramāsa/Lunar Month	Phálgun (first half)
Karma/action and Kāraka/significations	Acts of self-promotion (fame, mass media, etc.), artistic performances, visual presentations, protection of wealth, performance of black magic, climatic disturbances, threats to colonies (epidemics/pandemics/contamination)
Devata/Deity	Bhaga: one of twelve Ādityas, brother to Uṣas (first light)
Pooja/ceremonial items	White and red flowers, Palasha (*Butea monosperma*) and Karaveera (*Nerium oleander*), Garuda (eagle), red sandalwood, Bilwa wood (*Aegle marmelos*) incense
Ahuti/Fire ritual	Cooked chickpeas, mustard seeds and Priyangu (*Callicarpa microphylla*) cast into fire 108 times with Gāyatrī mantra
Nakshatrayoga	Those offering rice and ghee on the day of this star attain happiness and prosperity

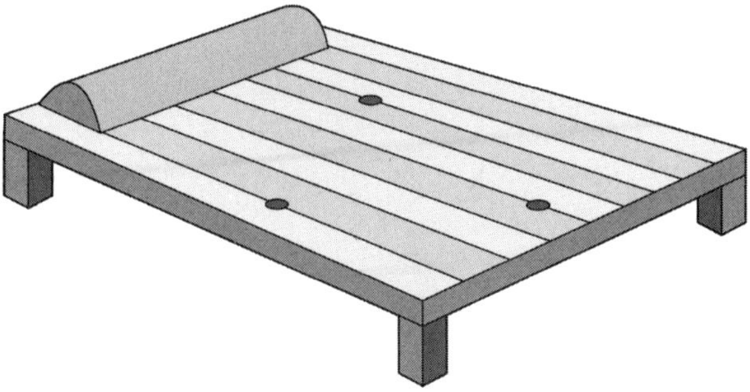

12. Uttaraphalguni

Sinhala	Utrapal
Tārā/Stars	β and 93 Leonis
Rashi/Sign	26° 40' Leo – 10° 00' Virgo
Chinha/Symbol	Cot or hammock
Gaṇa/Temperament	Human
Jāta/Sex	Masculine
Ruling Planet	Sun
Dosha	Vāta
Shakti	Patronage
Maha Guna	Sattva
Varna/Caste	Warrior
Chāndramāsa/Lunar Month	Phálgun (second half)
Karma/action and Kāraka/significations	Throne rooms, temples, boundaries of colonies, marriages, education, economics (money-making), leadership, agriculture, entering a new home, planting herbs, taking sustenance (nurturing), treatment of diseases, auspicious Nakshatra for performing mantra and other religious rituals
Devata/Deity	Aryaman: one of twelve Ādityas and devotee of Sûrya (Sun)
Pooja/ceremonial items	Plaksha (*Ficus uliginosa*), blue lotus (*Nymphaea caerulea*), red cloth, sindoora (red lead/cinnabar), Zatacchada (Indian woodpecker[32]) red rice, Guggulu or mustard seeds
Ahuti/Fire ritual	Badara (*Ziziphus mauritiana*) or Priyangu (*Callicarpa microphylla*) cast into fire 108 times with Gāyatrī mantra
Nakshatrayoga	Offerings of navara[33] rice and ghee on the day of this star make one honoured in heaven

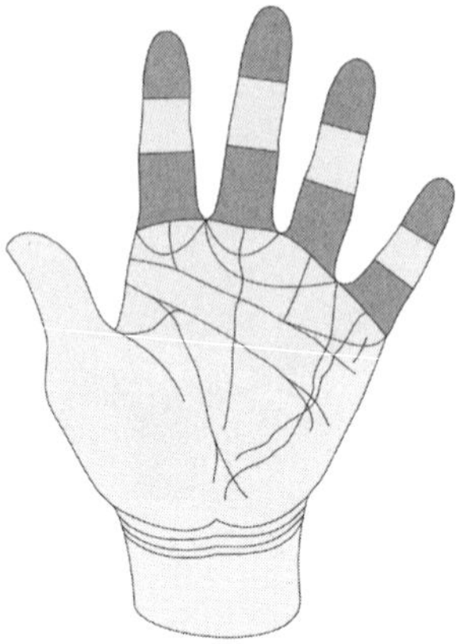

13. Hastā

Sinhala	Hatha
Tārā/Stars	δ, γ, ε, α, β and η Corvi
Rashi/Sign	10° 00' – 23° 20' Virgo
Chinha/Symbol	Hand
Gaṇa/Temperament	Divine
Jāta/Sex	Feminine
Ruling Planet	Mercury
Dosha	Vāta
Shakti	Inventive
Maha Guna	Rajas
Varna/Caste	Merchant
Chāndramāsa/Lunar Month	Chaitra (first third)
Karma/action and Kāraka/significations	Empowering gemstones, Hastā Rekha Shāstra, Jyotish, magic, massage therapy, preparation (grinding) of herbs, Hastā/Paṇi Grahanam[34] (taking of the hand), travel, leadership, new vehicles, new homes, jewels, establishing new kingdoms
Devata/Deity	Savitar: one of twelve Ādityas, charged with the conveyance of souls into the afterlife
Pooja/ceremonial items	Red cloth, red flowers, red sandalwood, Plaksha (*Ficus uliginosa*), Amratakan (*Spondias pinnata*), Śuka Pakshi or Raktapada (parrot), golden statue of Sûrya, Dashanga Guggulu (a mixture of ten aromatic resins/gums) for incense purposes
Ahuti/Fire ritual	Wheat flour and jaggery pudding, cast into fire 108 times with Gāyatrī mantra
Nakshatrayoga	One obtains worldly bliss offering a horse or elephant on the day of this star

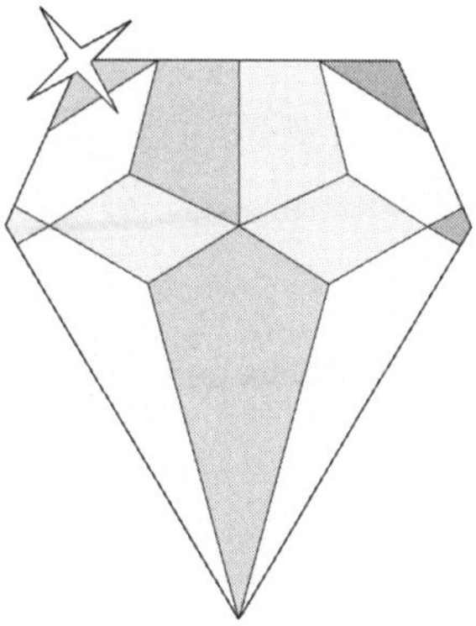

14. Chitrā

Sinhala	Sitha
Tārā/Stars	α and ζ Virginis
Rashi/Sign	23° 20' Virgo – 6° 40' Libra
Chinha/Symbol	A jewel or pearl
Gaṇa/Temperament	Demon
Jāta/Sex	Feminine
Ruling Planet	Mars
Dosha	Pitta
Shakti	Creating
Maha Guna	Tamas
Varna/Caste	Farmer
Chāndramāsa/Lunar Month	Chaitra (middle third)
Karma/action and Kāraka/significations	Planting herbs, landscaping (ornamental gardens), architecture, engineering, construction of yantra, wearing of astrological pendants, acquisition of jewels, mining gemstones, Vedic studies, learning, Hastā-mudrā (ritual hand gestures), painting, graphic design, marriage, purchasing or tending elephants and horses
Devata/Deity	Twastar: artificer to the gods, given the title Viśvarūpa (omniform) for his ability to manifest all manner of beings by will alone
Pooja/ceremonial items	Multicoloured cloth, ornaments, jewels, white objects, Bilwa (*Aegle marmelos*), Baka (crane), golden statue of Twastar, saffron, sandalwood, multicoloured flowers, wheat flower and jaggery cooked as a pudding, Shala niryasa (*Shorea robusta*) aromatic resin incense
Ahuti/Fire ritual	Chitrānna[35] (flavoured rice), cast into fire 108 times with Gāyatrī mantra
Nakshatrayoga	Perfumery offered on the day of this star grant access to the celestial gardens in which maidens dance and play

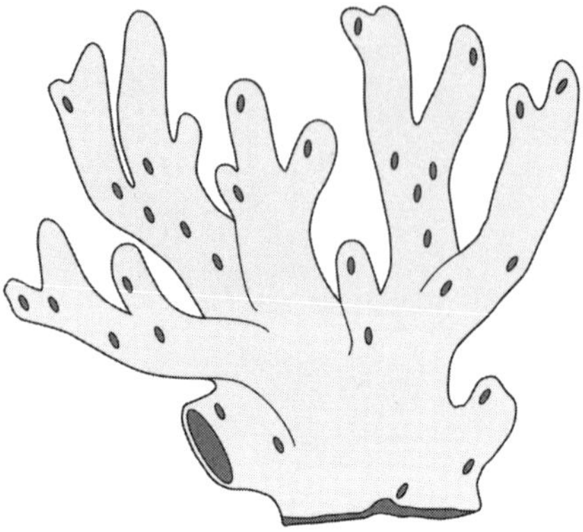

15. Swati

Sinhala	Saa
Tārā/Stars	α and ε Bootis
Rashi/Sign	6° 40' – 20° 00' Libra
Chinha/Symbol	Coral or sword
Gaṇa/Temperament	Divine
Jāta/Sex	Masculine
Ruling Planet	Rāhu
Dosha	Kapha
Shakti	Self-reliance
Maha Guna	Tamas
Varna/Caste	Butcher
Chāndramāsa/Lunar Month	Chaitra (final third)
Karma/action and Kāraka/significations	Harvesting medicinal plants, tending botanical gardens and leisure parks, treatment of disease, Jyotish, Rasa Shāstra (alchemy), work that requires precision (making pillars for temples), swiftness, flexibility, riding in chariots, education, studying for exams, women in fifth month of pregnancy, Yajnopaveeta (sacred thread ritual)
Devata/Deity	Vāyu: personification of the wind, as distinguished from Vāta (dosha). Vāyu was an important deity in Rig Veda, commonly evoked as the dual deity Indrā-Vāyu
Pooja/ceremonial items	Ornaments, red cloth (ruby red), Garuda (eagle) Arjuna (*Terminalia arjuna*), black eagle wood or sandalwood incense, golden statue of Vāyu
Ahuti/Fire ritual	Laaja (puffed) rice, cast into fire 108 times with Gāyatrī mantra
Nakshatrayoga	Alms of any sort given on the day of this star are renowned to grant benefits and reward

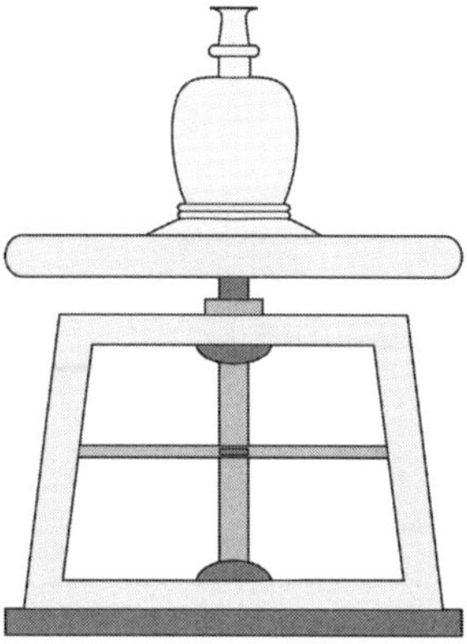

16. Vishaka

Sinhala	Visaa
Tārā/Stars	ι, α, β and σ Libræ
Rashi/Sign	20° 00' Libra – 3° 20' Scorpio
Chinha/Symbol	Potter's wheel or archway
Gaṇa/Temperament	Demon
Jāta/Sex	Masculine
Ruling Planet	Jupiter
Dosha	Kapha
Shakti	Star of purpose
Maha Guna	Rajas
Varna/Caste	Outcaste
Chāndramāsa/Lunar Month	Vaishāka (first half)
Karma/action and Kāraka/significations	Spiritual practice, gemstone cutting and wearing, taking medicine, healing/therapies, overcoming diseases, seasonal agriculture, harvesting, digging wells and the constructing water tanks
Devata/Deity	Indrā-Agnī: most venerated of all dualistic deities, many exhalant hymns are given in praise of Indrā-Agnī (Vedic warrior gods)
Pooja/ceremonial items	Kapitha[36] (*Limonia acidissima*), Ulūka (owl), golden statue of Indrā-Agnī, oil of Devadaru (*Cedrus deodara*) for incense, Shatapatri (rose petals), red saffron, wheat flour and jaggery pudding
Ahuti/Fire ritual	Milk rice sweetened with jaggery, cast into fire 108 times with Gāyatrī mantra
Nakshatrayoga	Those offering diamonds, cattle, milk or ghee on the day of this star attain heaven

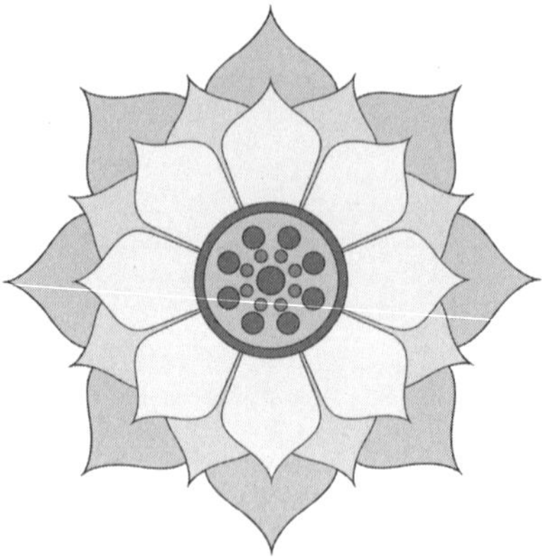

17. Anuradha

Sinhala	Anura
Tārā/Stars	δ, β1/β2 and π Scorpii
Rashi/Sign	3° 20' – 16° 40' Scorpio
Chinha/Symbol	Lotus flower
Gaṇa/Temperament	Divine
Jāta/Sex	Feminine
Ruling Planet	Saturn
Dosha	Pitta
Shakti	Success
Maha Guna	Tamas
Varna/Caste	Śūdra
Chāndramāsa/Lunar Month	Vaishāka (second half)
Karma/action and Kāraka/significations	Yogic practice, mantra, developing Siddhī (supernatural powers) diagnosis of disease (root causes), manufacture of medicine, testing gold and gemstones, purchasing vehicles, collecting animal horns, acquisition of cows, bulls and elephants, safe journeys and long lasting marriages
Devata/Deity	Mitra: known as a sustainer of gods, his role appears mostly supportive, stabilising the space between the Earth, Sun and heavens
Pooja/ceremonial items	Red cloth, Panasa/Jackfruit (*Artocarpus heterophyllus*), Śuka Pakshi or Raktapada (parrot), golden statue of Mitra, lotus flowers, Sabji (red banana flower), Bilwa wood incense
Ahuti/Fire ritual	Red milk rice sweetened with jaggery, cast into fire 108 times with Gāyatrī mantra
Nakshatrayoga	Those giving clothes, fabric or rice on the day of this star are honoured in heaven for one hundred Yugas

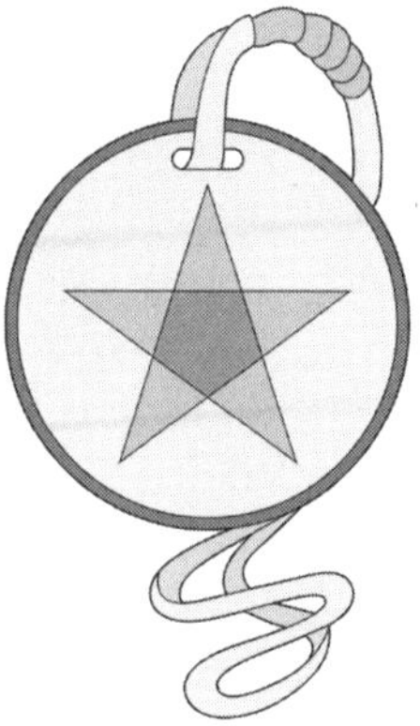

18. Jyestha

Sinhala	Deta
Tārā/Stars	α, σ and τ Scorpionis
Rashi/Sign	16° 40' – 30° Scorpio
Chinha/Symbol	Talisman, umbrella or earring
Gaṇa/Temperament	Demon
Jāta/Sex	Masculine
Ruling Planet	Mercury
Dosha	Vāta
Shakti	Vanquishing
Maha Guna	Sattva
Varna/Caste	Farmer
Chāndramāsa/Lunar Month	Jyestha (first half)
Karma/action and Kāraka/significations	Personal challenges, acts of faith, courage, affording protection to the weak or helpless, surgery, war, weapons, winning over opponents, conquering new lands, political gains, surrender, wild horses and elephants (stampeding out of control)
Devata/Deity	Indrā: primarily a thunder deity, Indra's secondary roles included dispelling darkness and the removal of drought through the liberation of rain
Pooja/ceremonial items	Betel nut tree (*Piper betel*), Kokila (Jacobin cuckoo), rice and sesame seeds (cooked), all yellow flowers, sandalwood, Pātala[37] (*Steriospermum suvaveolens*) or black eagle wood incense
Ahuti/Fire ritual	Chitrānna with ghee, cast into fire 108 times with Gāyatrī mantra
Nakshatrayoga	Those offering yams or green vegetables to a Brahmin on the day of this star realise all their wishes

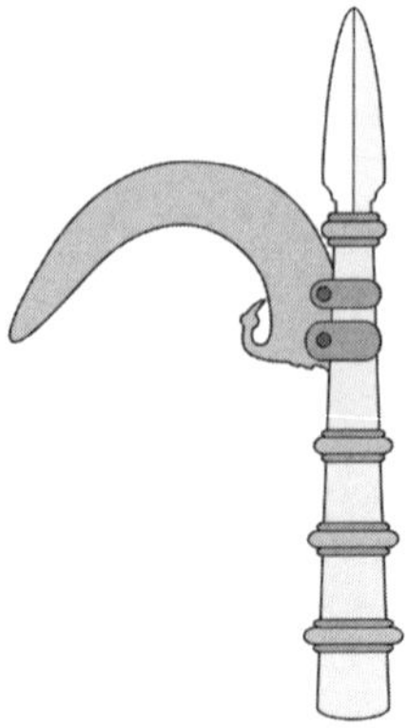

19. Mula

Sinhala	Mula
Tārā/Stars	λ, υ, ι, κ, θ and η Scorpionis
Rashi/Sign	0° – 13° 20' Sagittarius
Chinha/Symbol	Elephant goad, roots of a herb, lion's tail
Gaṇa/Temperament	Demon
Jāta/Sex	Masculine
Ruling Planet	Ketu
Dosha	Vāta
Shakti	Destructive
Maha Guna	Rajasic
Varna/Caste	Butcher
Chāndramāsa/Lunar Month	Jyestha (second half)
Karma/action and Kāraka/significations	Planting herbs, wholesome food (especially root vegetables), Jyotish, mantra, surgery, marriages, new homes, building Aushadhi (pharmacies) and pilgrimages
Devata/Deity	Niriti: guardian of the south west and daughter to Adharma (immorality) and Hiṃsā (violence), better known as the goddess of dissolution and destruction
Pooja/ceremonial items	Red cloth, black ornaments, climbing plants (creepers) or tubers, Chakra Vāka (brahmany duck),[38] black statue of Niriti, black gram cooked with red saffron and ghee, black eagle wood, blue louts flower, Ajasrnga (goat horn) / Salai Guggulu (*Boswellia serrata*) or Shala[39] (*Shorea robusta*) for burning/incense, sandalwood
Ahuti/Fire ritual	Black gram, fruits, sandalwood and flowers, cast into fire 108 times with Gāyatrī mantra
Nakshatrayoga	Offerings of roots or nuts to a Brahmin on the day of this star help pacify ones ancestors

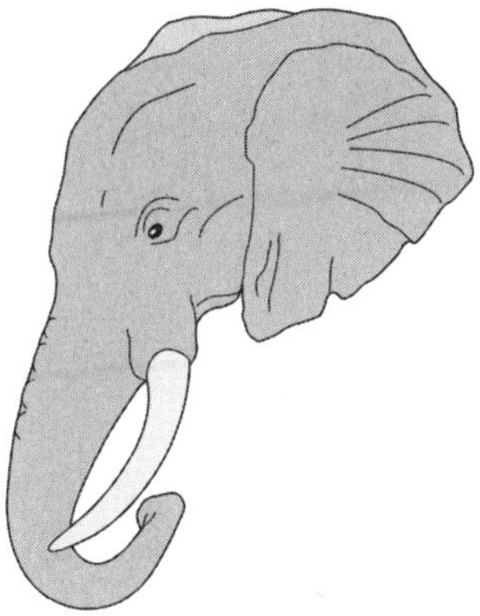

20. Purvashadha

Sinhala	Puwasala
Tārā/Stars	δ, ε, η and λ Sagittarii
Rashi/Sign	13° 20' – 26° 40' Sagittarius
Chinha/Symbol	Elephant tusk
Gaṇa/Temperament	Human
Jāta/Sex	Masculine
Ruling Planet	Venus
Dosha	Pitta
Shakti	Unsubdued
Maha Guna	Tamasic
Varna/Caste	Brahmin
Chāndramāsa/Lunar Month	Áshádha (first half)
Karma/action and Kāraka/significations	Hydrotherapy, agriculture, soil fertilisation, sowing seeds, deep wells, lakes, preparation of herbal remedies, Rasāyana therapies, use of protective mantra, Graha tantra[40] (demonology), weapons, training with weapons, Pitru Paksha
Devata/Deity	Apas: goddess of water and one of the eight Vasus in the service of Indrā
Pooja/ceremonial items	White cloth, Baka (crane), white sandalwood (Chandana[41]), Kaluva lotus (*Nelumbo nucifera*), Tintrini/tamarind (*Tamarindus indica*), Manasheela (realgar), Kankusta (*Garcinia cambogia*), rice, milk and brown sugar pudding
Ahuti/Fire ritual	Laaja and flowers, cast into fire 108 times with Gāyatrī mantra
Nakshatrayoga	Pots of curd given to Brahmin (after fasting), help one attain birth into a family owning many cows, on the day of this star

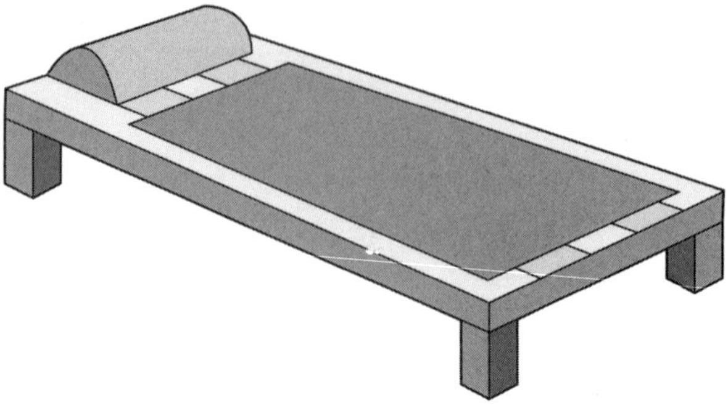

21. Uttarashadha

Sinhala	Uturusala
Tārā/Stars	σ, ζ and τ Sagittarii
Rashi/Sign	26° 40' Sagittarius – 10° 00' Capricorn
Chinha/Symbol	Wooden bed/cot
Gaṇa/Temperament	Human
Jāta/Sex	Masculine
Ruling Planet	Sun
Dosha	Kapha
Shakti	Victory
Maha Guna	Sattva
Varna/Caste	Warrior
Chāndramāsa/Lunar Month	Áshádha (second half)
Karma/action and Kāraka/significations	Planting/growing herbs, treatment of diseases, defeat of ones enemy, pilgrimages, education, gardens, plants and forests, divine worship, kings, rulers and leaders, anna prashana,[42] temples, auspicious undertakings
Devata/Deity	Vishvadevas: a collective of minor gods and goddesses that included Vasus, Ádityas, Rudras, Maruts, Aṅgirasas and Ṛbhus
Pooja/ceremonial items	White colour, white sandalwood, Pañca Varna Pushpa,[43] Kokila (Jacobin cuckoo), wood of Amla (*Emblica officinalis*), Pañca Bhakshya[44] (sweet bread), golden idol of Vishvadevas
Ahuti/Fire ritual	Rice and ghee, cast into fire 108 times with Gāyatrī mantra
Nakshatrayoga	When milk and ghee (sweetened with honey) are given to a wise man on the day of this star, the individual attains honours in heaven

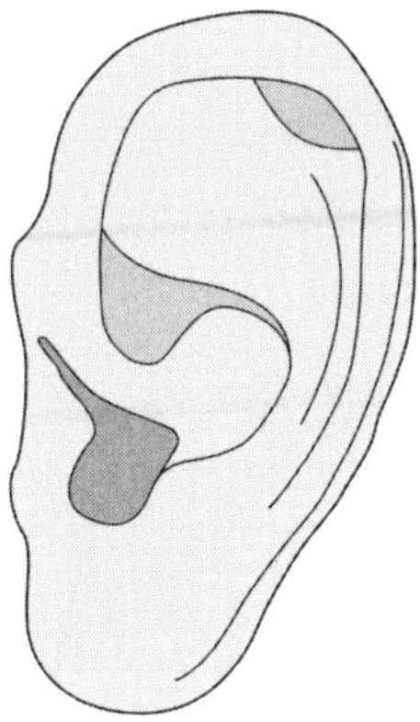

22. Śravana

Sinhala	Suwana
Tārā/Stars	α, β and γ Aquilae
Rashi/Sign	10° 00' – 23° 20' Capricorn
Chinha/Symbol	An ear or three footsteps
Gaṇa/Temperament	Divine
Jāta/Sex	Feminine
Ruling Planet	Moon
Dosha	Kapha
Shakti	Listening
Maha Guna	Rajas
Varna/Caste	Outcaste
Chāndramāsa/Lunar Month	Śravana (first third)
Karma/action and Kāraka/significations	Spiritual devotion, Yagya, pooja, Vrata (devotion), Nirāhāra (fasting), mantra, renunciation, initiation, making music, preparation of medicinal remedies (especially Rasāyana formulae), education, Gārbha-ādana,[45] ear piercing and Shanti-homam ritual
Devata/Deity	Vishnu: Vishnu means 'highest step'. His rulership over this star places considerable emphasis over its role within the asterisms. Vishnu is the second of three supreme divinities in Hinduism (collectively known as Trimūrti)
Pooja/ceremonial items	Black cloth, Aswatha (*Ficus religiosa*), Jala Kukkuti (black-headed gull), black statue of Vishnu, saffron, sandalwood, mustard seed, Tulsi (*Ocimum tenuiflorum*), red flowers, Dhashaga Guggulu (ten aromatic herbs), cooked shali rice cooked and offered with mantra to Vishnu, milk rice pudding made with red rice
Ahuti/Fire ritual	Aswatha wood and Lāja, cast into fire 108 times with Gāyatrī mantra
Nakshatrayoga	Those offering rugs or cloth on the day of this star are carried by white conveyances freely entering heaven

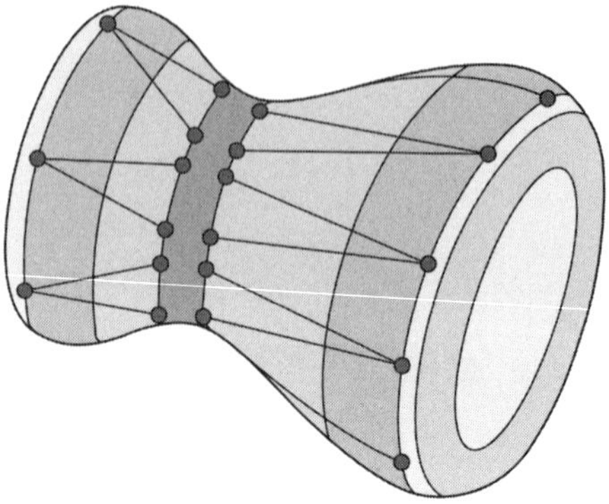

23. Dhanistha

Sinhala	Denata
Tārā/Stars	β, α, γ and δ Delphini
Rashi/Sign	23° 20' Capricorn – 6° 40' Aquarius
Chinha/Symbol	Two-headed drum
Gaṇa/Temperament	Demon
Jāta/Sex	Feminine
Ruling Planet	Mars
Dosha	Pitta
Shakti	Bringing renown
Maha Guna	Tamas
Varna/Caste	Farmer
Chāndramāsa/Lunar Month	Śravana (middle third)
Karma/action and Kāraka/significations	Wearing gemstones, Yajnopaveeta[46] (sacred thread), medicinal treatment (including surgery), burning, cutting and forging of metal, buying ornaments, vehicles or cloth, nourishment, building temples, royal courts, Upanayana Samskara[47] (acceptance ritual)
Devata/Deity	Vasus: a collective of eight important deities: Soma (Moon), Dharā (Earth), Anila (wind), Uṣas (dawn), Anala (fire), Dhṛuva (pole star), Pratyūsa (pre-dawn) and Parjanya (god of thunderstorms)
Pooja/ceremonial items	White cloth, white flowers, Tummeda (bumble bee), golden statue of the Vasus, sandalwood, Jati/jasmine flowers (*Jasminum grandiflorum*), Guggulu, Sûrya maṇḍala, wood of the fig tree, mung beans, red rice and aromatic flowers
Ahuti/Fire ritual	Milk and jaggery, cast into fire 108 times with Gāyatrī mantra
Nakshatrayoga	Those offering clothes, fabrics or cattle on the day of this star are eligible to freely enter heaven

24. Shatabhishak

Sinhala	Siyawasa
Tārā/Stars	λ, τ, δ, η, ζ, γ and α Aquarii
Rashi/Sign	6° 40' – 20° 00' Aquarius
Chinha/Symbol	Lotus, wheel, basket of herbs
Gaṇa/Temperament	Demon
Jāta/Sex	Feminine
Ruling Planet	Rāhu
Dosha	Vāta
Shakti	Healing, veiling
Maha Guna	Sattva
Varna/Caste	Butcher
Chāndramāsa/Lunar Month	Śravana (final third)
Karma/action and Kāraka/significations	Āyurveda/rasāyana therapies, visha shodhana (purification of poison), such as narcotic/hallucinogenic herbs, alchemy/Rasa Shāstra, digging of wells, walled gardens, agriculture, travel, gemstones and coral, collections, marriages, charity and the training of horses
Devata/Deity	Varuna: a powerful oceanic deity featuring prominently in early Vedic poems
Pooja/ceremonial items	Red cloth, khadira (*Acacia catechu*), Kokila (Jacobin cuckoo), golden statue of Varuna, malayaja sandalwood,[48] blue lotus, ghee and Guggulu incense, Māṃsa (meat of deer or goat) offered to fire,[49] puja with offerings of honey and ghee
Ahuti/Fire ritual	Rice milk pudding and white flowers, cast into fire 108 times with Gāyatrī mantra
Nakshatrayoga	Offerings of aloe or sandalwood made on the day of this star aid one to abide in the Deva realm

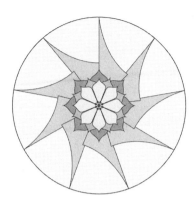

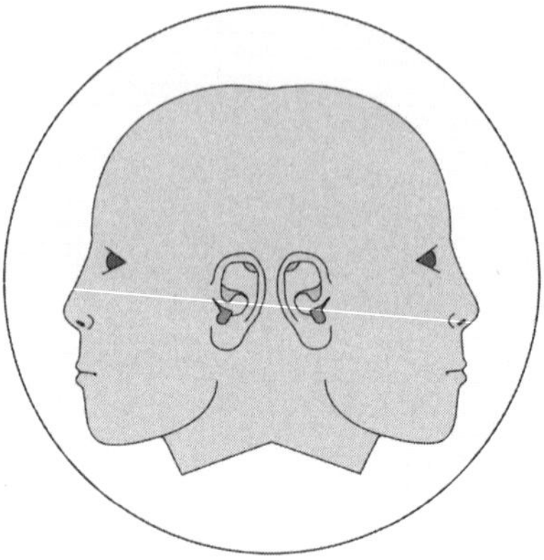

25. Purvabhadra

Sinhala	Puwaputupa
Tārā/Stars	α and β Pegasi
Rashi/Sign	20° 00' Aquarius – 3° 20' Pisces
Chinha/Symbol	Two-faced man
Gaṇa/Temperament	Human
Jāta/Sex	Masculine
Ruling Planet	Jupiter
Dosha	Vāta
Shakti	Upraising
Maha Guna	Rajas
Varna/Caste	Brahmin
Chāndramāsa/Lunar Month	Bhádrapada (first third)
Karma/action and Kāraka/significations	Education, cleansing with salt water, Vamana (vomiting), gemstone purification, sacred mantra, use herbal medicines, digging of wells, construction, agriculture/irrigation, planting herbs, construction of yantra, tantric practices, removing enemies and gambling
Devata/Deity	Aja-ekapād: meaning 'single-footed goat' – perhaps connected to a number of aerial/storm deities such as Rudra or Ahi-budhnya
Pooja/ceremonial items	Black cloth, Shamali (*Salmalia malabarica*[50]), Kapota (pigeon), golden statue of Aja-ekapād, red saffron, Arka (*Calotropis gigantea*), Guggulu (incense), cooked rice, yoghurt and flowers
Ahuti/Fire ritual	Kushmanda (ash pumpkin) and ghee, cast into fire 108 times with Gāyatrī mantra
Nakshatrayoga	Those offering coins on the day of this star obtain much bliss

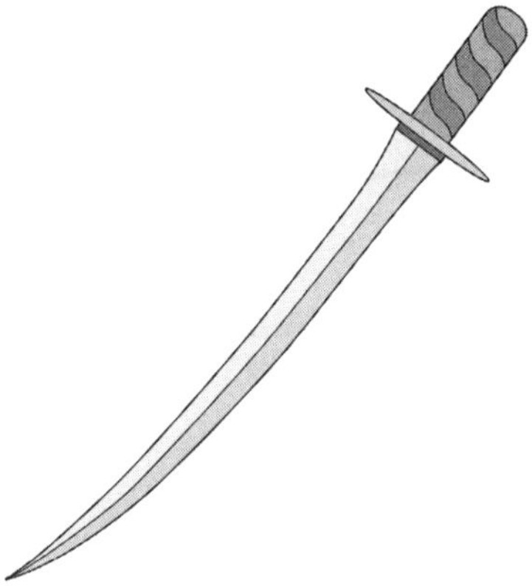

26. Uttarabhadra

Sinhala	Utraputupa
Tārā/Stars	α Andromedae and γ Pegasi
Rashi/Sign	3° 20' – 16° 40' Pisces
Chinha/Symbol	Sword or sea monster
Gaṇa/Temperament	Human
Jāta/Sex	Feminine
Ruling Planet	Saturn
Dosha	Pitta
Shakti	Warrior
Maha Guna	Tamas
Varna/Caste	Brahmin
Chāndramāsa/Lunar Month	Bhádrapada (second third)
Karma/action and Kāraka/significations	Worship of deities, construction of sacred buildings, construction of yantra, planting herbs, potentising gems, sculptures, marriages, fire rituals, wearing new clothes
Devata/Deity	Ahi-budhnya: thought to be inspired by a particular form of atmospheric phenomena, detailed description of its form is lacking. Ahi-budhnya is sometimes referred to as a serpent in the depths
Pooja/ceremonial items	White cloth, Pichumanda (neem wood[51]), Ulūka (owl), golden statue of Ahi-budhnya, white flowers, rose flower, Barbara (wild basil), Guggulu and ghee (incense)
Ahuti/Fire ritual	Cooked rice, jaggery and milk, cast into fire 108 times with Gāyatrī mantra
Nakshatrayoga	Those offering mutton on the day of this star bring pleasure to the Manes (progenitors)

27. Revati

Sinhala	Rawathi
Tārā/Stars	ζ, ε and δ Piscium
Rashi/Sign	16° 40' – 30° Pisces
Chinha/Symbol	Fish or drum
Gaṇa/Temperament	Divine
Jāta/Sex	Feminine
Ruling Planet	Mercury
Dosha	Kapha
Shakti	Wealth bringer
Maha Guna	Sattva
Varna/Caste	Śūdra
Chāndramāsa/Lunar Month	Bhádrapada (final third)
Karma/action and Kāraka/significations	Jyotish, deity worship, consecration of yantra, preparation of healing remedies, wearing gemstones, planting herbs, wearing of sacred thread, marriages, construction of sacred spaces (temples), acquiring horses or elephants
Devata/Deity	Pushan: one of twelve Ādityas, this deity was considered as overseer/protector of travellers and sustainer/guardian of cattle
Pooja/ceremonial items	Red cloth, butter tree (*Madhuca indica*), Myura (peacock), golden statue of Pūṣan, red saffron, Arka (*Calotropis gigantea*), Guggulu incense, Navadhana (nine types of grain[52]), cooked rice, saffron and red flowers
Ahuti/Fire ritual	Sesame, rice and fruits, cast into fire 108 times with Gāyatrī mantra
Nakshatrayoga	Those offering cattle or pots of milk on the day of this star are granted safe passage to all lands

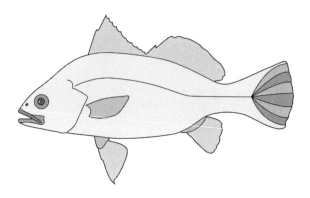

Chapter 11

HEALTH AND NAKSHATRAS

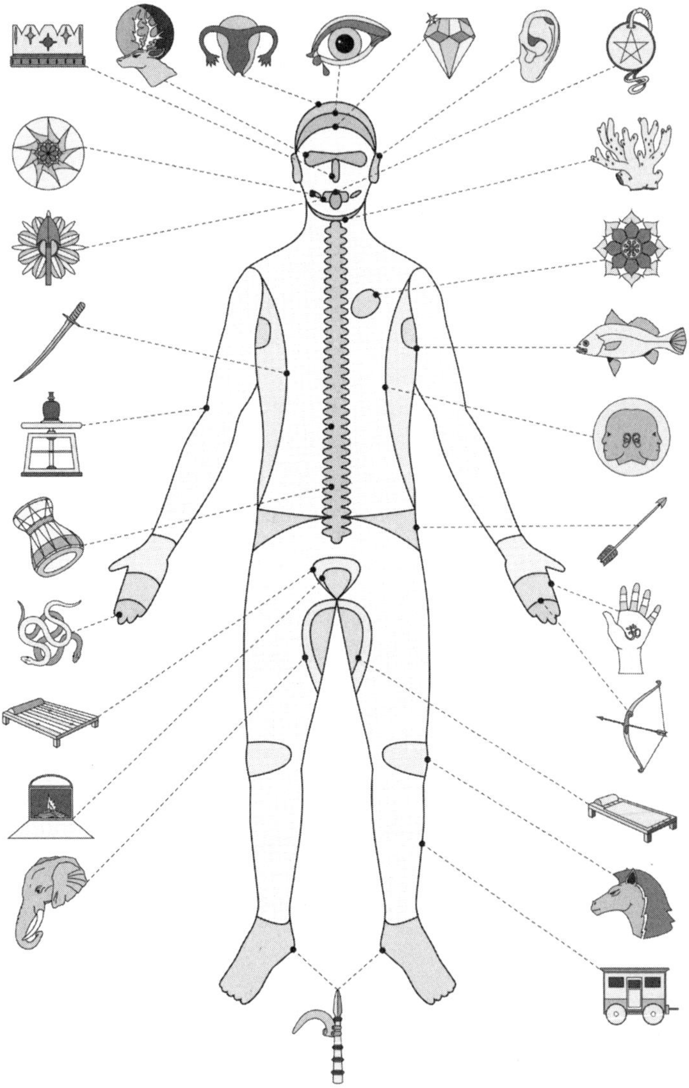

The Cosmic Man (Nakshatra Puruṣa) as described in Vāmana Purāṇa.

References to Nakshatra Puruṣa are to be found in Purāṇic texts (notably *Vāmana* and *Matsya Purāṇa*). Little explanation of their origination is given, excepting to say: 'all constellations dwell within the body of Lord Krishna and in so worshipping these different body parts, one not only attains longevity (resistance to disease), but ultimately liberation.'

Whilst a number of Purāṇa detail *some* astronomical data on Nakshatras (such as *Garuda Purāṇa*), it is often with reference to their seasonal reappearance, that is, rituals timed to coincide with their rising, zenith or setting. Such rituals include an observance of one's progenitors, the coronation of kings, the performance of abhisheka (consecration of sacred idols), bathing in sacred rivers, sowing of seeds, harvesting of crops, construction of new homes/water tanks and the taming of wild animals – to name but a few!

Medical astrology almost exclusively gives precedence to zodiacal *solar* bodily associations over those of its lunar counterpart. The reasoning behind this hierarchy is Moon's 'appropriated' light from Sûrya, with which it then onwardly animates Nakshatras (fixed stars). However, this appropriate illumination was thought useful in highlighting 'subtleties' or underlying causes that distress bodily tissues – as the Moon rules the night, the subconscious and hidden things. As previously noted, all Nakshatra qualities translate to the palm. During hand analysis, the medical implications of Nakshatras should also be kept in mind, particularly when interacting with lines or symbols found tenanting their allotted positions.

Some connections between Nakshatras and health are explored in Table 11.1.

Table 11.1 Connections between Nakshatras and health

Nakshatras	Dosha	Body Part/s	Health Conditions
Ashwini	Vāta	Knees, head (cerebral hemispheres) and soles of feet	Higher instances of febrile states, injuries to the head (brain), meningitis, thrombosis, paralytic strokes, anaemia, muscle spasm (neuralgia), imbalances of VK dosha
Bharani	Pitta	Head (crown), face, pineal, pituitary and hypothalamus glands, eyes and toes	Intestinal infections, lack of beneficial gut-flora, accidents or injury to the neck and face, muscular spasm, connective tissue weaknesses
Krittika	Kapha	Waist, eyes, neck, larynx, tonsils and lower jaw	Prone to irregular elimination (constipation or bouts of diarrhoea), persistent fever,[53] lower back pain, inflammatory disorders, typhoid, stomach cramping, arthritis and insomnia

Rohini	Kapha	Shins, mouth, palate, tongue, cervical vertebrae and legs	Disturbed apana-vāyu (poor elimination), haemorrhoids, fistula, painful swellings about the breasts, injury to face and neck, irregular menses, sunstroke, high blood pressure, heart problems and persistent aching in calf muscles
Mrigashirsha	Pitta	Eyes, ears, tonsils, jugular vein vocal cords and thymus	Acid reflux and abdominal bloating, weak eyesight, skin allergies, paralysis, constipation, haemorrhoids, high blood pressure, heart disease and disorders of the blood
Ardra	Vāta	Hair (forelock), eyes, throat, shoulders and arms	Insufficient or irregular digestive capability (low agnī), diseases of the throat, weakness of arms and shoulders, poor hair growth, insomnia, asthma, cough, pneumonia and diseases arising from poor sexual habits
Punarvasu	Vāta	Fingers, ears, throat, shoulder blades, pancreas, liver and nose	Recurring digestive parasites, mal-absorption of minerals (digestive insufficiency), persistent fevers and headaches, weakness of the lungs and liver, pancreatic imbalance, inner ear sensitivities (vertigo), injury to the throat and shoulder blades
Pushya	Pitta	Mouth, lungs, stomach and ribs	Abdominal bloating, heaviness of the stomach and feelings of nausea, gastric ulcers, childhood asthma (weakness of the lungs), tuberculosis, jaundice, fevers and colic, pancreatic imbalances, injury to the ribs and mouth
Aslesha	Kapha	Fingertips, fingernails, oesophagus, stomach, diaphragm and pancreas	Poor circulation, fatigue, anaemia, digestive sensitivity, weakness of the oesophagus, diaphragm or pancreas, liver disease, dropsy, Vāta (moving pains), injury to the feet and hands, hard-to-diagnose ailments
Magha	Kapha	Nose, chin, lips, spine and spleen	Respiratory weakness, cardio arrhythmia, injury to the spinal cord (dorsal region), weakness of the spleen and kidneys, recurring rhinitis, sensitivity of the stomach/digestive tract and recurrent migraine headaches
Purvaphalguni	Pitta	Genitalia, inner thighs, lower spine and hips	Chest infections, asthma or shortness of breath, heart disease, abnormalities of the spinal cord, diseases of the genitals, high blood pressure, paralysis of limbs, asthma and persistent ulcers
Uttaraphalguni	Vāta	Genitalia, outer thighs, liver, intestines, bowels and navel	Sensitive skin, rosaceae, blisters, sores and itchiness, weakness of asti-dhātu (porosity of bone), thrombosis, shoulder pain, dysentery, bowel and liver complains, appendicitis, intestinal weakness, diseases of the genitals

Nakshatra	Dosha	Body Part/s	Health Conditions
Hastā	Vāta	Hands, small intestine, digestive enzymes and secreting glands	Poor water/sugar metabolisation (prameha/ diabetes, injury to the hands, constipation, IBS, diarrhoea, diseases of secreting glands, under production of digestive enzymes, ring worm
Chitrā	Pitta	Forehead, kidneys, lumbar vertebrae and neck	Vertigo (inner ear infections), hearing loss, tinnitus, injury to the forehead, kidney stones, brain fevers, diabetes, retention of urine, abdominal ulcers, appendicitis, hernia, sciatica (weakness in lumbar region of spine)
Swati	Kapha	Jaw and chin, teeth, skin, bladder and urethra	Weakness of vision, propensity to cataracts, *muscae volitantes* (floaters), skin ailments, weakness of the bladder and urethra, falling of teeth and kidney stones
Vishaka	Kapha	Arms, lower abdomen, pancreas, rectum, bladder and prostate gland	Ear damage, hearing loss, inflammation of the inner ear, vertigo, weakness of the arms, haemorrhoids, abdominal pain, weak kidneys, blockage of pancreatic ducts, bladder infections, enlarged prostate gland, bladder wall inflammation and uterine cysts
Anuradha	Pitta	Heart, nasal bones, pelvis, rectum and anus	Prone to sinusitis, rhinitis, nose bleeds, etc.; weakness of the bladder, genitals, rectum and pubic bone; chest infections, constipation, menses, piles and high fever
Jyestha	Vāta	Tongue, colon, ovaries, womb, genitals and anus	Diseases of mouth, gums and palate, including teeth, jaw and throat; weakness of the colon, anus, genitals, ovaries, womb and neck
Mula	Vāta	Feet, legs, lumbar vertebrae and sciatic nerve	Respiratory weakness, shortness of breath and pronounced chest infections; weakness of the hips, thighs, feet, stomach, eyes and mouth; sciatica, rheumatism or limb paralysis
Purvashadha	Pitta	Thighs, hips, arteries and veins	Weakness of kidney, water retention, urinary calculi; weakness of the thighs, hips, sacral region of the spine, iliac arteries, veins, lungs (respiration), heart and circulation; propensity toward gout
Uttarashadha	Kapha	Thighs, arteries, veins, knee joints and patella	Sensitive stomach, over-production of mucus, nausea; weakness of lymphatic vessels, knees, skin, ears, urinary system; dysentery, typhoid, allergies or eczema
Śravana	Kapha	Ears, lymphatic system, reproductive system, testes and ovaries	Loss of appetite, sensitive gums (mouth ulcers); weakness of lymphatic vessels, knees, skin, ears, urinary tract; dysentery, typhoid, allergies or eczema

Dhanistha	Pitta	Spine, cerebrospinal fluid, ankles and calf muscles	Damage to tendons/ligaments, rheumatic conditions; weakness of the lower back, liver, urinary tract; high blood pressure, neurosis, arthritis of knees and ankles, injury to the shins and the fracturing of leg bones
Shatabhishak	Vāta	Teeth, lower jaw, knees and ankles	Falling of teeth and hyper-acidity; diabetes, weakness of the calves, injury to the chin, bilious attacks, typhoid, high blood pressure, paralysis and high fevers
Purvabhadra	Vāta	Sides of torso, navel, ankles, feet and toes	Vitiated Kapha, over-production of mucus (chest); weakness of the lungs, mental trauma, rheumatism, liver complaints, constipation, swelling of the ankles, feet and toes
Uttarabhadra	Pitta	Sides of the torso, navel, ankles, feet, toes and toenails	Vitiated Vāta; cramps, muscular fatigue in the chest area; weakness of feet, lungs and teeth, associated with anaemia, fever, digestive irritability, constipation, piles and epilepsy
Revati	Kapha	Armpits, lymph system and feet	Prone to skin inflammation such as rashes, sores and boils; weakness of the feet and toes, congestive diseases of the chest, mental disorders, stomach ulcer, nephritis, lethargy, excessive bile production, genital diseases caused by excessive sexual indulgence

NOTES

1. Known in Śrī Laṇkā as Nekatha.
2. The diagram at the beginning of Chapter 7 gives an indication of the areas occupied by each Nakshatra. However, much like star constellations these positions may sometimes float – indications straying into adjacent Nakshatras.
3. Some calculations of Nakshatras used a 28th division called Abhijit (α lyra). This star has been included on the Nakshatra Divisions diagram for reference only, it has not been included in palm positions.
4. Due to the lunar orbital tilt, the daily motion of the Moon may appear less than constant.
5. Known also as the Sun's Pathways (Ravi-marga), this great circle is inclined to Earth's celestial equator by 23.5°. The word 'ecliptic' refers to it being the reference point for calculating solar and lunar eclipses.
6. In some cases two Yogatârâ fall into the same Nakshatra. It should be noted here that some discrepancies also exist with regard to the identification of certain Yogatârâ.
7. Situated in the astrological sign Taurus, marked by the Yogatârâ: α Tauri/Aldebaran.
8. This lunar tale later becomes the origin of consumption or Ojaksaya.
9. Though the Sun draws life from the soil, its overall action is drying and eventually depleting. Earth's fertility was assigned to the Moon, who counteracted and nourished the effects of a mildly malefic Sun.
10. Drugs that have a powerful anti-ageing effect on the tissues. Many times these drugs may contain alchemical ingredients – for more information see the author's previous work: *Rasa Shāstra: The Hidden Art of Medical Alchemy* (Mason 2014).
11. Purāṇic sources include: Garuda, Vāyu, Nārada and Agnī Purāṇas
12. Special thanks to Utkoor Yajna Narayana Purohit for his contribution to this section.
13. *Strychnos nux-vomica.*
14. *Santalum album.*
15. *Commiphora mukul* – also known as buffalo-eyed Guggulu.
16. *Phyllanthus emblica.*
17. *Aquilaria malaccensis*, also known as Agar wood or black eagle wood.
18. A means to attain merit.
19. *Nerium indicum.*
20. *Eugenia jambolana.*
21. *Cinnamomum tamala.*
22. *Boswellia serrata.*
23. Musk gland.
24. *Acacia catechu.*
25. *Datura stromonium.*
26. *Ficus religiosa.*
27. *Amaurornis phoenicurus.*
28. *Mesua ferrea*, also known as Cobra Saffron.
29. *Curcuma longa.*
30. Yearly festival honouring one's ancestors, forefathers and the progenitors of mankind. The Pitris are generally propitiated during the sixteen lunar days of Pitru Paksha, currently falling in the middle of the lunar month Bhádrapada.
31. Hindu wedding ceremony, in which the parents literally pass their daughter to the groom.

32. *Picus Bengalensis.*
33. Rice originating in the Kerala region of India, often favoured in ceremonial use.
34. Clasping of hands in a Hindu marriage ceremony.
35. A flavoursome rice dish from southern India containing mustard seeds, peanuts, curry leaves, lentils, garlic, mangoes, turmeric, etc.
36. Also known as wood apple or elephant apple.
37. Also known as Fragrant Rose Flower.
38. *Tadorna ferruginea.*
39. Agnivallabha – burns with ease.
40. Also known as Butavidya.
41. Highly aromatic form of sandalwood.
42. Feeding times for infants.
43. Five castes of flower.
44. Chick pea and kithul jaggery base for coconut, cardamom, poppy seeds and nutmeg, rolled inside bread.
45. Pre-pregnancy preparation to ensure strong and healthy progeny.
46. Sacred cotton thread tied with deer skin and awakened through Gāyatrī Mantra.
47. Literally, under the eyes of the teacher/guru.
48. Malaysian sandalwood.
49. Shatabhishak is a demon Nakshatra and so sometimes propitiated with the flesh of animals.
50. Also known as Rakta Pushpa (red silk cotton tree). Known to attract multiple forms of wildlife, this tree is favoured in Āyurveda for its blood-cleansing properties.
51. *Azadirachta indica.*
52. Wheat, rice, green gram, horse gram, chick peas, white beans, black sesame seeds, black gram and bengal gram.
53. The deity Agnī was the originator of fever; he was assigned the task of extinguishing human life by his manifestation of fevers.

PART V

UPAYAS (REMEDIAL MEASURES)

Chapter 12

REMEDIAL MEASURES (UPAYAS)

A physician should perform fire sacrifices and offer oblations on days specific to the seizure of patients by an evil spirit. Which ever is desired by that patient, i.e. bathing, clothes, fats, meats, wines, milk or jaggery should be given on such days. Offerings of precious gemstones, perfumes, garlands, grains, honey, ghee, etc. These are common/general procedures of treatment.

Aṣṭāñga Hṛdayam

Perhaps one of the most interesting and practical aspects of palmistry/astrology is its use of remedial measures. These are a variety of techniques designed to counteract or enhance planetary influences (known as *grahaprabhāv*). Having assessed the palm, an astrologer is almost certainly expected to advise on ways to promote or negate benefic (saumya) or malefic (krūra) glances, issued from planets and known as *graha-dṛṣṭi* (Graha = planet and dṛṣṭi = sight).

There are many tried and tested remedies from which to choose; however, the degree to which an individual is prepared to participate in the remedy will play an important part in its success. It should at all times be kept in mind that you cannot simply buy your way out of karma, but at the same time some avenues of appeasement are not without cost. Primary gemstones, such as those outlined in the next section, are almost always going to be expensive; however, there are excellent substitute gems or alternative methods of influencing the planets, and all of these should be explored before resorting to highly expensive options.

Across the board, yantra are one of the most effective methods of placating unruly planets. However, these inevitably require *sampark*, that is to say, a means by which they 'connect' to a particular planet, so each yantra must first be attuned to the planet/s in question.

The following presents a number of popular upaya for readers' consideration and experimentation! For more information on yantra see Chapter 14.

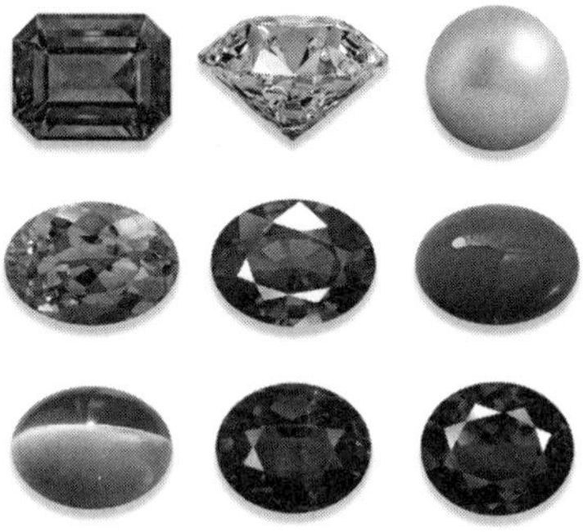

Gemstones (Maṇi) from top left to bottom right: Emerald (Mercury), Diamond (Venus), Pearl (Moon), Topaz (Jupiter), Ruby (Sun), Red Coral (Mars), Cat's Eye (Ketu), Blue Sapphire (Saturn) and Garnet (Rāhu).

GEMSTONES (MAṆI)

> The lord (Vishnu) holds the two-fold divisions of egotism, namely elements and organs of sense in the shape of his conch shell and bow. In his hand a discus, representing the mind which is the strength of all and that which in flight, excels the speed of the wind. Holder of a mace, his vaijayenti (garland) contains pañcamaharatna[1] (five precious gemstones), i.e. pearl, ruby, emerald, sapphire and diamond – each a symbol of the five great elements.
>
> *Vishnu Purāṇa*

Astrological remedies (on the whole) seem unduly biased in their use of gemstones in alleviating or enhancing the effects of planets, yet collectively classical works on Vedic Astrology exhibit a decided lack of detail in regard to *ratnadhāraṇa* (wearing gemstones for astrological purposes). Esteemed works such as *Arthashāstra,*[2] *Garuda Puṛanā,*[3] and *Brihat Saṃhitā,*[4] while recounting their supernatural origin, caste, ruling deity[5] or relating signs of genuineness, fail to connect gems with planet.

Brihat Parasara Hora Shāstra[6] (a compendium of rediscovered astrological scriptures) considers gems 'fortune bestowing', that is to say, likely to manifest themselves during a particular planetary period, saying: 'During the planetary period of Venus one sees gains in white clothes, conveyances, gemstones (such as pearls), beautiful damsels, etc.' Here too, this work makes no specific correlation between a particular planet and gemstone.[7]

References to 'planetary gemstones' are to be found in India's alchemical[8] literature, which does acknowledge an affinity between planet, gem and metal in a medicinal capacity.[9] For example, *Rasaratna Samuccaya*[10] promotes *mudrādhṛtam*, gemstones set within rings for bodily adornment. These are said to gain planetary blessings. However, associations between specific gems and planets are a little different from those now commonly adhered too.

This in part may be due to earlier medicinal categories merging with later astrological considerations. Alchemical texts, by and large, are more preoccupied with the medicinal grade of a gemstone as bhasma.[11] Bhasmas are literally gems reduced to alchemical ash, believed useful in fixing or binding liquid mercury (Hg) to a cohesive state.

As time passed, alchemical literature began to expound on a planet/gem correlation, as well as the medicinal effects of gemstones to counteract the morbidities of certain planetary rays. *The Crested Jewel of the Rasa Lord* (Rasendracūḍāmaṇi), authored by Acharya Somadeva, appears as one of the earliest alchemical texts in this regard, its c.12th century AD texts directly connecting each planet with a particular gemstone.

MODERN APPROACHES

Contemporary astrological works fully embrace gemstones as remedial measures, unleashing a whole sway of astr-gem-aficionados, supplying a host of apotropaic stones. This is not to say that gemstones are without efficacy, far from it – I've known or heard of too many cases where gemstones worn to soothe planets turned the day around.

I would instead like to add a cautionary note on jewellers and lapidary, making the reader aware that these industries are not without peril to lay gem-seekers. Keep in mind always that even the experts can be fooled – so to be forewarned is to be forearmed. Knowing a trusted jeweller or gemmologist can be a great asset – and ALWAYS proceed with caution. Get purchases checked wherever possible.

PREPARING, SETTING, PAIRING AND WEARING OF GEMSTONES

The medicinal application of gemstones (known as Ratnachikitsa) is now an established approach amongst astrologers, seeking to alleviate less-than-favourable planetary fortune. Table 12.1 indicates some of the more popular recommendations for the selection, pairing and setting (metals) of newly acquired gemstones.

Table 12.1 Planets, gemstones and setting

Sun (fire)	Ruby (P) Sunstone (S) *Setting metal:* Gold/Silver	**Mars (fire)**	Red Coral (P) Red Spinel[12] Red Agate/ Carnelian(S) *Setting metal:* Silver	**Saturn (air)**	Blue Sapphire (P) Blue Amethyst (S) *Setting metal:* Iron/Stainless Steel/Silver
Respective Fingers	Ring Finger (right hand)	**Respective Fingers**	Ring Finger (right hand)	**Respective Fingers**	Middle Finger (right or left hand)
Moon (water)	Pearl (P) Moonstone (S) *Setting metal:* Silver/Gold	**Jupiter (water)**	Yellow Sapphire (P) Citrine or Topaz (S) *Setting metal:* Gold	**Rāhu (air)**	Hessonite[13] (P) *Setting metal:* Silver
Respective Fingers	Index Finger (left hand)	**Respective Fingers**	Index Finger (right hand)	**Respective Fingers**	Middle Finger (right or left hand)
Mercury (earth)	Emerald (P) Peridot (S) *Setting metal:* Silver/Platinum	**Venus (water)**	Diamond[14] (P) Clear Quartz (S) *Setting metal:* Silver/ Platinum	**Ketu (air)**	Chrysoberyl/ Cat's Eye (P) *Setting metal:* Silver
Respective Fingers	Little Finger (left or right hand)	**Respective Fingers**	Middle Finger or Little Finger (left hand)	**Respective Fingers**	Middle Finger (right or left hand)

(P) = primary stone; (S) = substitute stone

There is a whole set of do's and don'ts prior to wearing and after wearing new gemstones. Here for the reader's interest I have listed nine common guidelines that should be adhered to when taking the plunge and buying a planetary gemstone:

1. Gemstones should be pre-soaked for at least 12 hours in milk, saltwater or *pañcamrita* (five nectars[15]) prior to wearing.
2. All gemstones should be conically cut and set 'open-backed', so as to fully contact skin.

3. All gemstones are ideally set in either gold or silver (see Table 12.1).
4. Gems are typically worn on finger, wrists or about the neck.
5. Gemstones may be worn for long periods; however, their effect may not materialise instantaneously with set levels of intensity. It is therefore recommended that a 'trial period' is initiated before dedicated wearing. Sleeping with the gemstone (under a pillow) is sometimes a good place to start, carefully noting changes in circumstance.
6. Gemstones exhibiting fracture/s or opaque spots after being worn for some period are said to indicate 'karmic stress' and are to be discarded. The idea here is that a gem has done its job, literally absorbing particularly virulent planetary rays which might have manifested to the wearer's misfortune. This 'shocking' proved too much for a stone, partially obscuring or shattering its structure.
7. Gemstones with unhappy histories, that is, those stolen or recovered (found without purchase), are likely to carry bad luck, so should be avoided.
8. Gems emitting a foul smell are to be avoided.
9. Irradiated, heat-treated or dyed gemstones are to be avoided.

HEALTH BENEFITS OF GEMSTONES

Table 12.2 outlines potential health benefits of gemstones, applicable to their associated planet.

Table 12.2 Health benefits of gemstones

Sun (Sûrya)	Ruby (P) Sunstone (S)	Gives strength to heart and nerves, improves circulation, digestion and vision. Promotes intellect, self-esteem and independence. Increases Pitta, reduces Kapha and Vāta
Moon (Chandra)	Pearl[16] (P) Moonstone (S)	Gives strength to heart and eyes, reduces hot emotions. Promotes kidney and bladder functionality, general rasāyana for bodily secretions/fluids. Pearls purify blood and reduce acidity. Increases Kapha, cools Pitta and reduces Vāta
Mars (Kuja)	Red Coral (P) Spinel/Agate/ Carnelian[17] (S)	Gives strength to respiratory and reproductive system. Coral nourishes blood, promotes strong connective tissue, promotes strong connective tissue, muscular strength and tendon elasticity. Reduces inflammatory conditions (cooling energetic). Increases Kapha, balances Pitta and reduces Vāta

Mercury (Budha)	Emerald (P) Peridot (S)	Rasāyana for nervous and respiratory systems, reduces inflammation, fevers, itching and skin complaints (loss of lustre). Useful in cases of eczema and asthma, improves attentiveness in children, tonifies blood. Emeralds promote homeostasis of Rasa Dhātu and support nervous tissue. Emeralds increase Kapha, reduce Pitta and Vāta
Jupiter (Brihaspati)	Yellow Sapphire (P) Citrine/Topaz (S)	Gives strength to eyes, teeth and gums. Balances hormonal/glandular system and supports the immune system. Yellow sapphire is warming, nutritive and builds tissue. It promotes digestion, strengthens hepatic functioning and is beneficial in cases of hearing loss and vertigo, it also aids in the absorption of minerals. Increases Kapha, reduces Vāta and slightly increases Pitta
Venus (Shukra)	Diamond (P) Herkimer Diamond/Clear Quartz (S)	Diamond has excellent anti-visha properties, it promotes longevity and strengthens Ojas.[18] Useful is cases of urogenital diseases, diabetes and weak pancreatic functionality. Diamond improves kidney functionality, boosts immunity and balances water metabolism, also has aphrodisiac properties. Increases Kapha, reduces Vāta and Pitta
Saturn (Shani)	Blue Sapphire (P) Blue Amethyst (S)	Blue sapphire reduces oedema, soothes painful joints and heals fractures (binds damaged tissue), promotes flexibility and reduces inflammation. Useful in cases of constipation, piles, varicose veins, poor circulation, paralysis, reduced vision, hearing loss and vertigo. This gemstone is generally considered to promote longevity. Increases Vāta and reduces Pitta and Kapha
Rāhu (North Node)	Garnet/Cinnamon Stone (P)	Garnet soothes nerves, reduces depression, allays fears and protects against external negative forces, increases appetite and promotes vitality, is generally known to promote prosperity and success, but also likely to encourage addiction of one sort or another. Increases Pitta, reduces Vāta and slightly increases Kapha
Ketu (South Node)	Chrysoberyl/Cat's Eye (P)	Chrysoberyl strengthens the immune system, protects against external pathogens, accidents and injury. It also helps reduce inflammation, paralysis and tonifies the nervous system. Cat's eye promotes astrological/occult power and psychic ability. Increases Pitta and Vāta while reducing Kapha

THE LEGEND OF BALA AND GEMSTONES

Garuda Puṛanā identifies the demon Bala[19] as the origin of gemstones, who after enduring eons of gruelling *sādhanā*[20] attained a boon from Lord Brahmā, who unwittingly granted him unbridled strength. Quickly defeating all competitors, he set about subjugating heaven and Earth.

Although tyrannical, Bala pledged 'unconditional' support for all necessary sacrifices, thereby ushering in his own demise. Skilfully crafting a sacrifice in honour of his inauguration, the gods remained vague as to the details of the service, but at the hour of need announced it was none other than the lord and heaven himself. Tricked into offering his body, the demon capitulated and was willingly slayed. His lifeless body then transformed into a resplendent gemstone. Fighting over the prize, the gods inadvertently shattered the great gem, whose pieces fell from the heavens, to be washed from the mountain tops by rain and rivers.

Variations of gemstone were attributed to parts of the former demon's body. Ruby (mānikya) became associated with the blood of Bala; it pacified dosha and protected the body from all manner of diseases. Pearls (moti), originating from the teeth of the once great demon, warding off all manner of evil, including poison. Wearing emerald brought victory in battle against any foe; emerald (tarksya) was derived from Bala's bile. Topaz (pushparaga) was derived from his skin and removed sterility from women, crowning them with maternity. Diamonds (hiraka) of all colours were considered the most effulgent and precious of stones; each still contained a particle of the demon. Diamonds were also associated with the bones of Bala. Blue Sapphire (nilama) was associated with the eyes of Bala. These gems were highly praised by the learned and said to be found on the foreshores of the sea of Śrī Laṇkā. Cat's Eye (vaiduryam) was formed from the resounding war-cry of the demon, forming subtle clouds of various colour before solidifying. Fossil crab-stone (*Karketana*) was associated with the claws of Bala, promising long life, healthy progeny and a mind free of evil thought. Quartz (bhismapaśana[21]) was derived from the semen of Bala and provided immunity from poison and attack from wild beasts; its wearer also enjoyed any number of wives. Realgar[22] (pulaka) was also associated with the claws of Bala, bringing wealth and progeny (darker variations of this stone were known to bring death upon those who kept it in their possession). From the demon's complexion came Blood-stone (raktapaśana), known to increase wealth and provide one with many servants. Finally, Red Coral (pravala) was derived from the entrails of the demon; its wearer enjoyed riches and was safeguarded from all manner of poisons and evil.

Chapter 13

METAL (DHĀTU)

> The learned have designated the planets as Sûrya (Sun), Chandra (Moon), Kuja (Mars), Budha (Mercury), Brihaspati (Jupiter), Shukra (Venus), Shani (Saturn), Rāhu and Ketu (ascending and descending lunar nodes). Their respective malignant influences entail the wearing of swarna (gold), rajata (silver), loha (iron), parādabandha (bound mercury), chandanam (pasted sandalwood), sphatika (rock crystal), naga (lead), pittala (brass) and kansya (bronze) by persons struck with them, on their bodies.
>
> *Garuda Purāṇa*

Metals, like gemstones, were also considered to have apotropaic powers, offering an important connection to planets. Indeed, direct association between metal and planet seems historically to have been well-established. It is not entirely clear when this connection had been made, but it is possible that adept metal-workers, over time, had catalogued working peculiarities unique to each metal. It was perhaps these peculiarities that later inspired the qualities now commonly attributable to planets via their associated metals. This idea is explored in the section 'Properties of Metal' later in this chapter.

SEVEN TISSUES (SAPTA DHĀTU)

Within the context of Āyurveda, another type of *Dhātu* related to bodily tissues is often translated to mean 'that which supports'. Sapta Dhātu[23] (or seven vital tissues) are a series of complex and specialised transformative 'membranes'. These were imagined to preside over different stages of the digestive process, each essential to the overall maintenance and healthcare of the body.

When we partake of food, chewing kicks off a series of internal alchemical processes, initiating a transformative process of gross to subtle. At each stage of digestion, some level of filtration/refinement of this transitory food mass takes place, before passing its remainder along. Subsequent Dhātus perform ever-advanced levels of processing, until only the most subtle of elements remain. These final few drops of 'rarefied food matter' are considered highly potent – so much so that they ultimately feed the procreative seventh tissue, which promotes new life (see Table 13.1).

Table 13.1 Sapta Dhātu*

1st level	Rasa	Plasma/lymph (clear part of blood)	Mercury (mercury)
2nd level	Rakta	Hgb/haemoglobin (red part of blood)	Moon (silver)
3rd level	Māṃsa	Muscle tissue/ligaments	Mars (iron)
4th level	Medas	Fat tissue/adipose (loose connective tissue)	Jupiter (tin)
5th level	Asthi	Bones/joints	Sun (gold)
6th level	Majjā	Brain tissue/marrow and nerve tissue	Saturn (lead)
7th level	Śukra	Semen/ovum (reproductive fluids)	Venus (copper)

* Sapta Dhātu have no direct equivalent in modern medicine, yet some correspondences may be useful for identifying tissues associated with this digestive process.

The ancients intuited this whole process to be carried out simultaneously, on three separate levels, namely:

- *Dhātu Transformation:* Here each of the seven tissues cook and transform nutrient material into a medium that can be accepted and digested by each subsequent Dhātu. The analogy is given of milk being transformed into curd, butter, then finally ghee.

- *Dhātu Transmission:* This witnesses each Dhātu filling to capacity then overflowing, like an elaborately tiered irrigation system. The expanding nutrient slowly filters down through each tissue, nourishing each upon contact.

- *Dhātu Selectivity:* This sees nutrients pass freely between all tissues, systematically harvested for essential content (relative to each Dhātu). The analogy of seeds and grains being feasted upon by different birds is often used. Each bird, having taken its fill, retreats to its nesting ground.

The whole process of digestion from start to finish was thought to correspond to a period of 708 hours or 29.5 days (roughly a synodic lunar month). This forms an important connection not only to the lunar cycle, but additionally connects each tissue to one of the seven planets and (by association) its corresponding metal (see Table 13.1).

PROPERTIES OF METAL

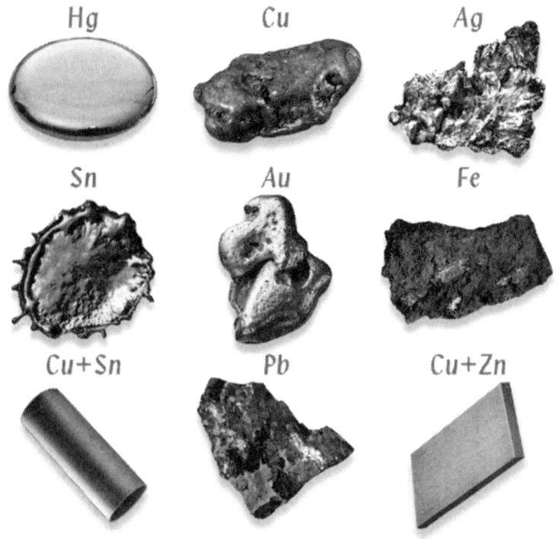

Metals from top left to bottom right: Hg/mercury (Mercury), Cu/copper (Venus), Ag/silver (Moon), Sn/tin (Jupiter), Au/gold (Sun), Fe/iron (Mars), Cu+Sn/bronze (Ketu), Pb/lead (Saturn) and Cu+Zn/brass (Rāhu).

Vedic Alchemy (Rasa Shāstra) categorises metal into a number of groups: liquid mercury (pārada), precious or pure metals (sudha[24]), ferrous or non-ferrous metals (puti[25]) and alloys (misra[26]). Additionally, metals were distinguished by hierarchy/caste (see 'Planetary Portraits' in Chapter 5). Here, gold and silver are deemed incorruptible 'royal' metals.[27] Tin, copper and zinc are of priestly caste. Iron is of warrior caste, while lead and the remaining alloys were of servile caste.[28]

Planet Mercury's namesake (Hg) is considered beyond caste, in as much as it forms an amalgam (mercury alloy) with a number of metals and minerals. Although planet Mercury is of royal blood (see 'Planetary Portraits' in Chapter 5), the unique properties of his metal place it in a venerated category, having the ability to transmute lower metals into higher states – such as gold, generally agreed to be the highest state any metal could attain.

Table 13.2 details some of the remedial benefits of metal as both medicine and talisman.

Table 13.2 Metal attributes

Sun/Gold (Au)	Considered an ageless metal, gold is without blemish, perfected and sattvic. Noted to have a heating quality (stimulating Pitta dosha), its taste is initially astringent, bitter and finally sweet. Gold gives strength to the heart, bones and joints, it is beneficial for the eyes (vision), and promotes courage. Its ability to remain untarnished confers longevity and wisdom upon its wearer
Moon/Silver (Ag)	Silver is also without blemish, ageless and representative of cooling 'feminine' energy, increasing Kapha dosha. It too has sattvic qualities. Its tastes are sour, astringent and sweet, its essence is oily and lekhana[29] (scraping). Silver reduces Vāta and Pitta, improving digestion by healing the stomach and gastric mucosa. It gives strength to the respiratory system and nourishes the eyes (improving vision). Silver counteracts the effects of poison, is aphrodisiac and rasāyana for mind and body
***Venus/Copper (Cu)**	Although subject to oxidisation, copper is considered sudha but also has tamasic qualities. The tastes of copper are astringent, bitter and sweet. It is heavy, heating, a little oily and scraping in nature. Copper reduces Kapha and Pitta, digesting fat while improving mobility and elasticity of tissues. Copper is anti-bacterial and anti-fungal (kills pathogens), it promotes vision, has emetic properties (counteracts the effects of poisoning). Incorrectly processed, copper is itself a poison
Mars/Iron (Fe)	Although subject to oxidisation, iron is considered sudha but also has rajasic qualities. The tastes of iron are astringent, bitter and sweet, initially cooling, with some accrued heating properties. Iron reduces Kapha and Pitta, it is drying and heavy, promoting healthy formation of blood. Iron destroys anaemia, strengthens the spleen and gives lustre to the skin. Iron counteracts the effect of poisoning, is aphrodisiac and a rasāyana for blood. Known as 'The Marshal of Metals', iron installs the will to succeed and the love of victory.
***Mercury/Mercury (Hg)**	Unique amongst metals, Pārada is considered vāhana (vehicle) for many metals; it has rajasic qualities. Pārada is Shad-rasa (having all six tastes), it is strongly heating. Its solidification is achieved by forming an amalgam with gold, silver, copper, lead, tin or zinc. United with sulphur, mercury converts to a stable black sulphide called kajjali. This combination is frequently used to produce pottali,[30] a semi-metallic ball of mercuric sulphide. Pottali may be worn as a talisman or ground to produce an internal medicine. Incorrectly processed, mercury can be highly toxic
***Jupiter/Tin (Sn)**	Tin is considered puti (a non-ferrous and fetid metal); it has rajasic qualities. The tastes of tin are bitter and astringent, it reduces Kapha but aggravates Vāta (its long-term effect is drying). Tin promotes intelligence, heals skin diseases, soothes the urogenital system, is an esteemed remedy in the destruction of diabetes, anaemia, vertigo, hearing loss, auto-immune conditions and digestive instability. Low levels of tin can manifest as nerve sensitivity, hair loss, hearing loss, depression and low self-esteem, with an increase in bone porosity

***Yasada/Venus/ Jupiter/Zinc (Zn)**	Zinc is considered puti (a non-ferrous and fetid metal); it has rajasic qualities. The tastes of zinc are bitter yet sweet and cooling in post-digestion. Zinc promotes healthy vision, strong teeth and bones, nourishes majjā dhātu (nerves and higher brain functioning) and also gives bala (strength). Low levels of zinc in the body usually manifest as pancreatic imbalances, depression, throat infections, inflammation, ulcers, bruises, stomatitis, low immunity (reduced ojas and low libido). Zinc and tin have similar properties; both have a low melting point and both resemble mercury (Hg) when heated. Rulership of zinc is jointly administered by Jupiter and Venus, favouring the attributes of the latter. Zinc is known to be a later addition to the planetary metals
***Saturn/Lead (Pb)**	Lead is considered puti; it has tamasic qualities. The tastes of lead are initially bitter then sweet; it is heavy, greasy and is heating in the long term. Lead promotes digestive strength, healthy joints and the elimination of toxins; it also has aphrodisiac properties. It is favoured in the treatment of auto-immune diseases, such as rheumatoid arthritis and eczema, inflammation in the urogenital system and useful in the treatment of diabetes. Lead reduces Vāta and Kapha but aggravates Pitta. It is referred to as Nāgā (snake) due to the hissing sound it produces when being processed. Incorrectly processed, lead can be highly toxic, accumulating in the brain, nervous system and kidneys
*** Rāhu/Brass (Cu+Zn)**	Brass is considered mishra (mixed); it has tamasic qualities. The tastes of brass are bitter, cold and drying, reducing Pitta and Kapha, but increasing Vāta. Brass promotes liver function and healthy blood, it is a hepatic rasāyana. Beneficial for the spleen, circulatory system and skin, the cleaning and scraping action of brass helps remove Āma (undigested food), parasites and accumulated dosha. Brass is considered an important yoga vāhin (vehicle) for other alchemical remedies. Incorrectly processed, brass can be toxic
*** Ketu/Bronze (Cu+Sn)**	Bronze is considered mishra (mixed); it has tamasic qualities. The tastes of bronze are bitter and pungent, its action is heating and lightening. Bronze reduces Pitta but aggravates Vāta with prolonged use. Bronze promotes strong vision, blood purity, gives hepatic/ digestive strength, removes toxins, kills intestinal parasites and reduces inflammation. Bronze has excellent anti-bacterial properties. Incorrectly processed, brass can be toxic

* Metals showing toxic properties, used only after stringent purification practices.

Chapter 14

YANTRA/TALISMAN

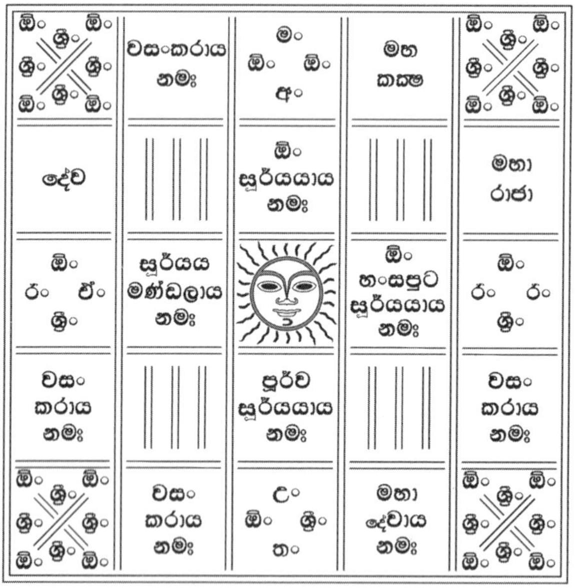

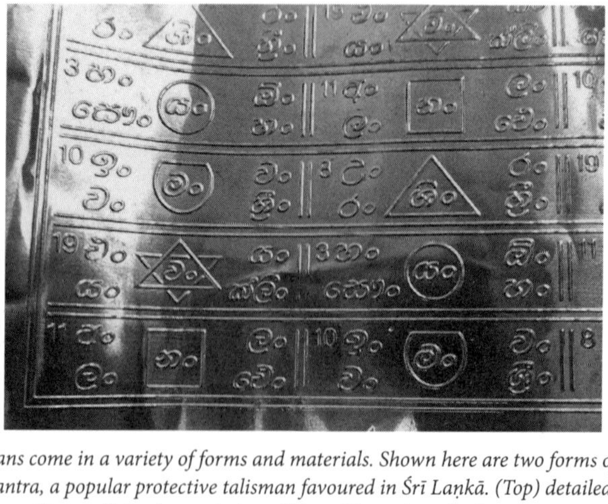

Talismans come in a variety of forms and materials. Shown here are two forms of Sûrya (Sun) Yantra, a popular protective talisman favoured in Śrī Laṇkā. (Top) detailed graphic for Sûrya Yantra, (below) a variation of Sûrya Yantra inscribed on thin copper sheet.

Yantra[31] in the form of astrological amulets are commonplace in Asia, especially in Śrī Laṇkā. I cannot remember meeting anyone who didn't wear some variation of necklace, bracelet, charm or ring, each skilfully manufactured to counteract negative astrological effects. Many Āyurvedic doctors I met on the island preferred to wear a nine-gem set (called Navaratna) as rings or pendants, and all reported having gained positive benefit from adherence to their astrologer's prescription.

The word *yantra* simply means a device or apparatus of varying complexity, usually based on specific geometric or numerological design. Yantra aim to reproduce a three-dimensional, inanimate (energetic) object, upon a two-dimensional surface. Yantras feature heavily in the many Hindu/Tantric rituals where involvement of a higher cosmic force is required. Yantra designs are varied and complex, with many variations on a theme. Whether constructed for ritualistic or talismanic purposes, yantra appear to be the preferred technology for negating or empowering planets. Their availability and reliability have made them highly desirable in astrological prescriptions. To their inscriber, yantra denote a consecrated area where the presence of a deity could literally be made to reside during ceremonial use. Indeed, the very act of yantra creation is considered a kind of visual meditation, bonding inscriber and deity into the energetics of the design.

Most astrological yantra prescribed by Śrī Laṇkān astrologers favour Buddhist themes, these focusing primarily on the removal of negative planetary forces. Their designs are exquisitely detailed and laboured over for many hours by a local shaman (medicine man). Although there is some scope for personal stylisation, most remain faithful to prescribed designs. A number of rules are to be adhered to whilst preparing yantra, for example:

- Yantra should not have crossing lines in their design as these disrupt the flow of energy. The empty spaces between the lines focus and hold energy.
- Yantra usually contain an individual's name, adding specificity to the overall design.
- Yantra are given sight (dṛṣṭi) and consecrated to a specific god (deva) or demon (yaksha). Most astrological yantra are in alignment to auspicious planets; however, inauspicious planets may also be favoured if they happen to represent a threat to health or vitality. In the case of the latter, planets are suitably restrained within the protective design of the yantra.
- Yantra should be awakened through offerings aligned to the deva concerned; for example, consecrations conducted during daylight

with flowers, milk, scented water or fruits favour benefic forces. Yantra honouring demonic forces may be consecrated after sunset with offerings of black cloth, animal blood or putrid foods.

- Favourable conditions are sought before potentising yantra. These include selecting a day or time favourable to the planet being honoured.
- During manufacture, appropriate mantra should be offered to the planet concerned – this will further empower its effects. Yantra should always be constructed with the good of the patient in mind.

(*Note:* I have given more detailed information on the use of yantra in my previous book, *Jyotish: The Art of Vedic Astrology* (Mason 2017). In my opinion, yantra are a great way to work with planetary energetics.)

SURAYA

Suraya are manufactured from a number of metals, including gold, silver and brass. They are available in a number of decorative forms, worn vertically (top) or horizontally (bottom).

Suraya[32] or astrological pendants are a popular means of adorning yantra (seeking to ward off negative planetary effects), often taking the form of horizontal or vertical tubes. These are commonly fashioned from brass, silver and gold. Copper yantra are then rolled and stored safely inside. Typically, the thin copper sheets bearing the inscriptions are smeared with an astrological oil, which is not only aromatic but serves to protect the copper from humidity and oxidation. Contents of Suraya can include yantra, gemstone ashes (bhasma) or dried herbs, each specifically targeted to entice or ward off planetary forces.

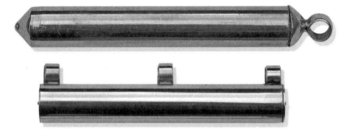

Chapter 15

CHARMED THREAD (PIRITHNOOLA)

Pirithnoola,[33] or charmed (cotton) thread, is a popular Śrī Laṇkā talisman. Commonly worn for protective purposes, it may be plain white or in some cases dyed with saffron or turmeric, producing a pleasing yellow/ orange hue.

Worn about the right wrist or upper arm, threads are to be replaced should they fray or fall. Pirithnoola are not worn continuously for more than a week. Replacement nool may be requested from Buddhist monasteries, where resident monks prepare them by chanting onto large balls of stringed cotton at sunrise and sunset.

Pirith refers to the rhythmic (*sutta*[34]) chants placed upon noola. Most pertinent to this section on Upaya is *nawagraha-shanthiya* or nine-planet pacification, a protective mantra calling upon planets to avert *graha-apala* (malefic rays) protecting against *avāsanāva* (bad luck).[35] Pirithnoola are thought to embody a promise, which at some point later in time the wearer dutifully honours, payment in kind for the protection afforded by the Grahas.

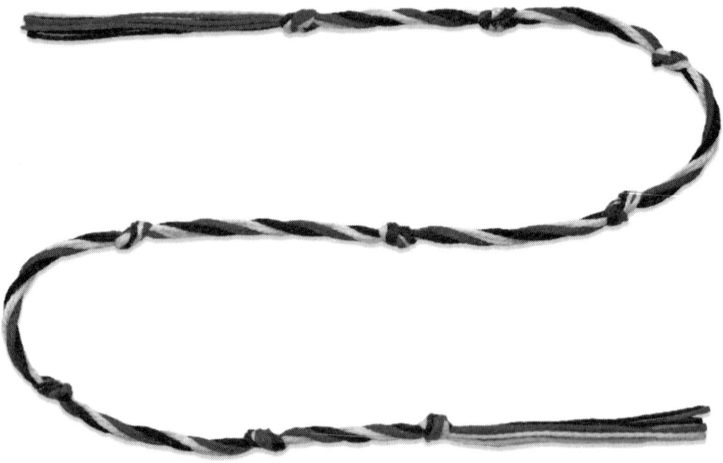

Sample of Śrī Laṇkān Cappota-nool or nine-knot charmed thread.

One variation of sacred thread (known as *Cappota-nool*) deals more specifically with planetary intervention and is issued by *Kapu-rala* (locally respected/wise person). The complexities of this particular thread (its manufacture and wearing) have been outlined in the following.

1. Construction of nine-knot thread:

- The distance between the tip of the middle finger and elbow (approx 18 inches) is covered three times by one thread.
- Three threads are used, their colours red, black and white.
- The total lengths of thread is now nine.
- The nine lengths are now interwoven or twined about one another and secured by nine equally disposed knots (representing the nine planets).
- The numerology is now: $3 \times 3 = 9$ (individual) and $3 \times 3 = 9$ (collective), $9 + 9 = 18$ $(1 + 8 = 9)$.
- Knots are left loose to capture planets or entangle malefic spirits.

2. Empowerment of nine-knot thread:

- The thread is energised by ritual. A banana leaf is cut and decorated by five coconut lamps, one at each corner and one in the middle. This makeshift altar is then decorated with five flowers of varying colour. Flowers of Ariconut (*Areca catechu*) are placed at the centre of the banana leaf. The empowerment ritual is commenced just before or just after sunset.

- The thread is empowered by chanting the mantra below, 108 times on Saturdays only. The patient is asked to be relieved of planetary afflictions. Prayers to Buddha may also be used.
- Capotta-nool should be removed at crossroads, graveyards, slaughter houses or in the company of women undergoing menses. Wearers should refrain from eating pork, eggs or dried fish.

Both types of noola are popular in Śrī Laṇkā and worn by a large number of its populace.

ආරක්ෂා මන්ත්‍රය (තෙල්, නූල්, හඳුන් මතුරා දෙනු)

ඕ අන්දිමාන මේ ප්‍රෙත කාමේ මෛත්‍රිෂණ දෙවියෙක් ක්‍රිෂණා දෙවියෙක් මුලෂුපයෙන් අද මේ නීච කපාල නම් තිත්තපට පාර ගැසී නම් තැවී නම් තවදියෙදිකරං කලසුල්ලාගේ තංකල ගෝමිය කට බැඳ ගතිං අත්දි මායා අන්දි භූපති අන්දිරාම අන්දි ප්‍රේමා අන්දිමා පෞලී අන්දිමාසො ගිනි අන්දිමා ඊශ්වර වාදේ ඕං ධාස් පීස් රමන රාමාදී ඔලාගිල් ඩිල් පට්ටියහං ත්‍රිහා ඕ හල් ද්‍රිඩයා නමඃ ඕං හ්රිං ද්‍රෝං ඔරුදු ග්‍රිෂට රාම යා දිට්ඝ සෝගිනියා යටහන් නමඃ ඕං හ්රිං රහිතං ග්‍රිදේස් අන්දි මාරාමයන් අන්දිම ක්‍රිෂටයා ඕං රාමයාත් ඕං ප්‍රෙතකාම අන්දිමේ පුඩා සෝමා අන්දිමේ රාලලදා නෙත් දුනු දියල සුරල්ලා බාඳගතිං ඔඕ යානාස් අංපස් අල්ලා දල්ලා ලල්ලා ඕං හ්රීං අංපසු තුංකරගතිං ඕං හාදිස් ඩිල්ලා වංගිනී ධීරේ සෝමා මා ඕං යඃ

Ārakśa Mantraya

(Offering thread, oil and sandalwood then chanting)

om andhimāna may preta kāme maithreeśhana deviyek krishnā deviyek mūlaśhūpayen ada may neecha kapāla nam thithapata pāra gasie nam thavie nam thavadiyedikaran kalasullāge thankala gomiya kata bandha gathin andhi māya andi bhupathī andhirama andhi prema andhimā powlee andhimāso githi andhimā eshwara vāde ohm dhās pees ramana rāmādee olagil dill pattiyahum thriha oh hul dhridayā namah: ohm hreem, dhrōm orudu ghrishta rāma yā dhitgha soginiyā yatahaṇ namah: ohm hreem rahitam grideśh andhi mārāmayan andhima krishataya ohm rāmayāth ohm pretakāma andhime pūda soma andhime rālaladā neth dunu diyala surallā bhandagithin ohm yānās ampas allā dallā lallā ohm hreem ampasu thunkaragathin ohm hādhis dilla vanginie dheere soma mā ohm yah:

Perhaps one of the most popular esoteric remedies is mantra. Mantra are an important and very traditional remedy for inauspicious planets. Despite their having been closely guarded secrets in the past, the use of mantra (to alleviate suffering) is now more available to the west, due largely to a surge of interest in Vedic Palmistry and Astrology. I remember one teacher telling me 'never underestimate the power of mantra', and so with that in mind the following chapter includes a mantra for each of the nine planets, first in Sanskrit, then Roman script (complete with diacritic marks). A literal translation of each mantra has been provided at the end of each.

(*Note:* Shorter versions of planetary mantra have also been given, see 'Honouring Navagrahas' in Chapter 17.)

Chapter 16

SACRED SOUNDS (MANTRA)

Sûrya (Sun)

ॐ सप्ताश्वरथमारूढं प्रचंडं कश्यपात्मजम्
श्वेतपद्मधरंदेवं त्वां सूर्यम् प्रणमाम्यहम्

Auṃ saptāśvarathamārūḍhaṃ pracaṃḍaṃ kaśyapātmajam
śvetapadmadharaṃ devaṃ tvāṃ sūryam praṇamāmyaham

Translation:
Auṃ, I bow before the Sun, who carries a white lotus, the elevated and formidable son of Rishi Kaśyapa, whose chariot is pulled by seven horses.

Chandra (Moon)

ॐ दधिशंखतुषाराभं क्षीरोदार्णव संभवम् ।
नमामि शशिनम् सोमं शंभोर्मुकुटभूषणम् ॥

Auṃ dadhiśaṅkhatuṣārābhaṃ kṣīrodārṇava saṃbhavam
namāmi śaśinam somaṃ śaṃbhormukuṭabhūṣaṇam

Translation:
Auṃ, I bow before the one who is colour of conch, curd or snow, who sprang from the waves of the milky ocean, he who contains soma, the image of a hare and adorns the crown of lord Śiva.

Kuja (Mars)

ॐ धरणीगर्भसंभूतं विद्युत्कांचन सन्निभम्
कुमारं शक्तिहस्तंच मंगलं प्रणमाम्यहम्

Auṃ dharaṇīgarbhasaṃbhūtaṃ vidyutkāṃcana sannibham
kumāraṃ śaktihastaṃca maṅgalaṃ praṇamāmyaham

Translation:
Auṃ, I bow before Mars (the auspicious one), young prince, born of earths womb, luminous like golden lightning, spear handed son of Śiva.

Budha (Mercury)

ॐ प्रियंगु गुलिकाश्यामं रूपेणा प्रतिमं बुधम्
सौम्यं सत्वगुणोपेतं तं बुधं प्रणमाम्यहम्

Auṃ priyaṅgu gulikāśyāmaṃ rūpeṇā pratimaṃ budham
saumyaṃ satvaguṇopetaṃ taṃ budhaṃ praṇamāmyaham

Translation:
Auṃ, I bow before Mercury, wise, mild and full of sattva, who by appearance I liken to the darkened reflection of priyaṅgu[36] *seeds.*

Brihaspati (Jupiter)

ॐ देवानांच ॠषीणांच गुरुकांचन सन्निभम्
बुद्धिमन्तं त्रिलोकेशं तं नमामि बृहस्पतिम्

Auṃ devānāṃca ṛṣīṇāṃca gurukāṃcana sannibham
buddhimantaṃ trilokeśaṃ taṃ namāmi bṛhaspatim

Translation:
Auṃ, I bow to Jupiter, intelligent lord of three worlds, treasure-like, you are teacher to the gods and sages (ṛṣi).

Shukra (Venus)

ॐ हिमकुण्ड मृणालाभं दैत्यानां परमंगुरुम्
सर्वशास्त्र प्रवक्तारं भार्गवं प्रणमाम्यहम्

Auṃ himakuṇḍa mṛṇālābhaṃ daityānāṃ paramaṃgurum
sarvaśāstra pravaktāraṃ bhārgavaṃ praṇamāmyaham

Translation:
Auṃ, I bow down before venus (Bhārgava – descendant of Bhṛgu), expounder of all shāstras, highest guru of the demons (Daityas), who resembles the stalk of lotus, snowy white in colouration.

Shani (Saturn)

ॐ नीलाञ्जन समाभासं रविपुत्रं यमाग्रजम्
छाया मार्ताण्ड संभूतं तं नमामि शनेश्वरम्

Auṃ nīlāñjana samābhāsaṃ raviputraṃ yamāgrajam
chāyā mārtāṇḍa saṃbhūtaṃ taṃ namāmi śaneśvaram

Translation:
Auṃ, I bow to the calm lord, born of the Sun (Sūrya) and Chāyā (shadow), elder brother to Yama, son of the Sun, who has a lustre like black añjana.[37]

Rāhu (Northern Lunar Node)

ॐ अर्धकायम् महावीर्यम् चंद्रादित्य विमर्दनम्
सिंहिका गर्भ सम्भूतम् राहुं तं प्रणमाम्यहम्

Auṃ ardhakāyam mahāvīryam caṃdrāditya vimardanam
siṃhikā garbha sambhūtam rāhuṃ taṃ praṇamāmyaham

Translation:
Auṃ, I bow before Rāhu, born from the womb of Siṃhikā, who eclipses the Sun and Moon, who is of half-body, yet great in valour.

Ketu (Southern Lunar Node)

ॐ पलाश पुष्पसंकाशं तारकाग्रह मस्तकम्
रौद्रं रौद्रात्मकं घोरं तं केतुं प्रणमाम्यहम्

Auṃ palāśa puṣpasaṃkāśaṃ tārakāgraha mastakam
raudraṃ raudrātmakaṃ ghoraṃ taṃ ketuṃ praṇamāmyaham

Translation:
Auṃ, I bow before Ketu, terrifying and violent (like Rudra), who seizes the stars and causes the setting of heavenly bodies, he who has the appearance of palāśa.[38]

Chapter 17

DEVIYO-BANDANA (DEITY WORSHIP)

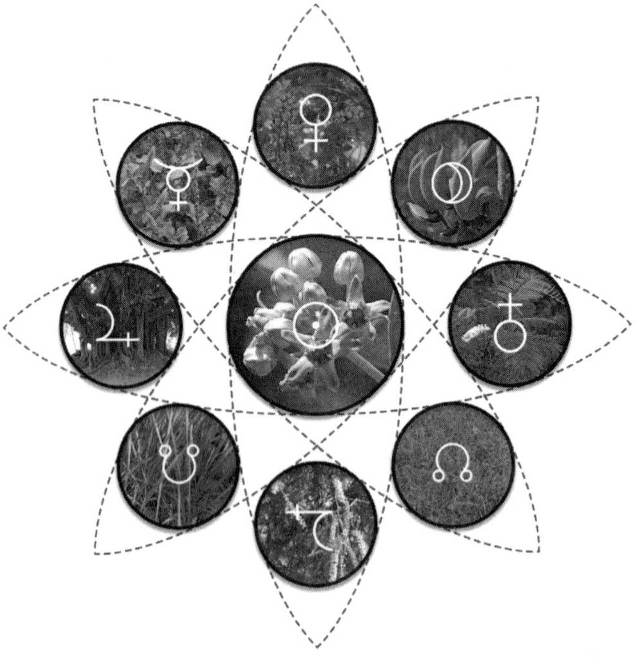

Navagraha Yantra or nine-planet configuration with associated planetary grasses/ plants/trees. Clockwise (from top): Venus – uḍumbara (Ficus racemosa), Moon – palasha (Butea monosperma), Mars – khadira (Acacia catechu), Rāhu – dūrvā grass (Cynodon dactylon), Saturn – shami (Prosopis cineraria), Ketu – kusha grass (Desmostachya bipinnata), Jupiter – aswatha (Ficus religiosa), Mercury – apamarga (Achyranthes aspera) and centrally, Sun – arka (Calotropis gigantea).

Āyurvedic classics such as *Caraka Saṃhitā, Susrutha Saṃhitā* and *Aṣṭāñga Hṛdayam* acknowledge and detail remedial measures as either corporeal (those actions which directly affect the body) or non-corporeal (those actions which seek to connect with higher non-physical sources, residing beyond the human senses). In greater detail these are:

- *Yukthi-vypashraya:*[39] Therapies that aim to re-balance the body through purification, tonification, diet/fasting, life-style exercise and medicines.
- *Satwa-avajaya:*[40] Therapies aiming to harmonise the mind, such as mantra, prayer, counselling, psychology and Deviyo-bandana, the latter seen to derive its effects through such techniques as yajna,[41] kratu,[42] bali,[43] homa[44] and ratnadhāraṇa.[45]

The following is an exploration of Deviyo-bandana, remedial measures that seek to propitiate the planetary deities.

HONOURING NAVAGRAHAS

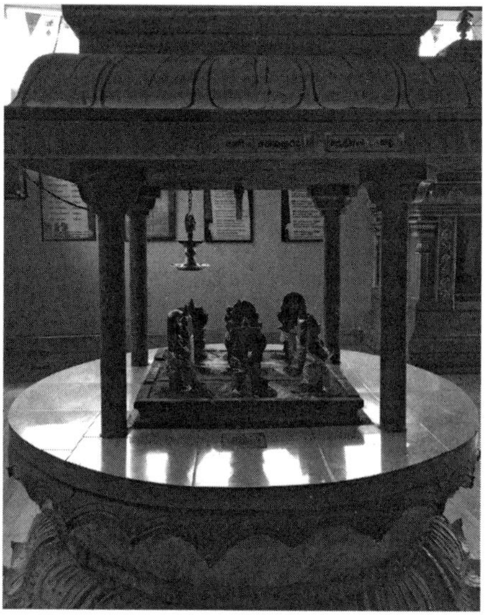

Nawagraha deities (Hindu Temple, Śrī Laṇkā).

After careful analysis of the palm, those proficient in Hastā Rekha should be able to offer a number of remedial measures to placate (or enhance) planetary emissions, diverting malefic forces while coercing benefic influences to deliver their bounties. The following outlines a number of commonly relied-upon actions and items advised in Deviyo-bandana.

Sûrya (Sun)	
Alternate name/s	Ravi, Vivasvant, Bháskara or Loka-chakshuh
Associated deity	Śiva, Agnī (Śiva = the destroyer, Agnī = fire god)
Gemstone	Ruby (primary), sunstone (substitute)
Metal	Gold (Au)
Colour	Red (scarlet)
Grain	Goduma dhanya (wheat)
Plant	Arka (*Calotropis gigantea*)
Sacred diagram	Vartulākāra Maṇḍala (circle)
Fasting	Sunday
Mantra	AUM SŪRYAYA NAMAHA or AUM GHRINI SŪRYAYA NAMAHA – chanted 108 times at sunrise on Sundays

Chandra (Moon)	
Alternate name/s	Soma, Indu, Nakshatra-nâtha or Śiva-sekhara
Associated deity	Parvatī (consort to Lord Śiva)
Gemstone	Pearl (primary), moonstone (substitute)
Metal	Silver (Ag)
Colour	White/pale blue
Grain	Tandula dhanya (paddy rice)
Plant	Palāśa (*Butea monosperma*)
Sacred diagram	Sama Caturasra Maṇḍala (square)
Fasting	Monday
Mantra	AUM SOM SOMAYA NAMAHA – chanted 108 times at sunrise on Monday

Kuja (Mars)	
Alternate name/s	Angáraka, Vakra, Rināntaka or Bhūmiputra
Associated deity	Kartikeya (god of war)
Gemstone	Red coral (primary), red spinel, red carnelian or red agate (substitute)
Metal	Iron (Fe)
Colour	Red (vermillion)
Grain	Kandulu dhanya (red gram)
Plant	Khadira (*Acacia catechu*)
Sacred diagram	Trikonākāra Maṇḍala (triangle)
Fasting	Tuesday
Mantra	AUM KUJAYA NAMAHA or AUM KRAN KRIN KRON SAH BHAUMAYA NAMAH – chanted 108 times at sunrise on Tuesday

Budha (Mercury)	
Alternate name/s	Saumya, Induputra, Jna or Bud
Associated deity	Vishnu (the preserver)
Gemstone	Emerald (primary), peridot (substitute)
Metal	Mercury (Hg)
Colour	Green
Grain	Mudga dhanya (green gram)
Plant	Apamarga (*Achyranthes aspera*)
Sacred diagram	Bānākāra Maṇḍala (arrow)
Fasting	Wednesday
Mantra	AUM BUDHAYA NAMAHA or AUM BRAN BRIN BRON SAH BUDHAYA NAMAH – chanted 108 times at sunrise on Wednesday

Brihaspati (Jupiter)	
Alternate name/s	Angira, Gīsh-pati, Suraguru or Guru
Associated deity	Indrā (king of the gods, wielder of lightning)
Gemstone	Yellow sapphire (primary), topaz/yellow citrine (substitute)
Metal	Tin (Sn)
Colour	Yellow
Grain	Chanaka dhanya (chickpea)
Plant	Aswatha (*Ficus religiosa*)
Sacred diagram	Ayatākāra Maṇḍala (rectangle)
Fasting	Thursdays
Mantra	AUM BRIM BRAHASPATYA NAMAHA – chanted 108 times at sunrise on Thursday

Shukra (Venus)	
Alternate name/s	Shodasānsu, Swetha, Bhṛiguja or Kāvya
Associated deity	Indrāni (consort to Indrā, queen of the gods)
Gemstone	Diamond (primary), clear quartz (substitute)
Metal	Copper (Cu)
Colour	White
Grain	Nishpava dhanya (Cowpea)
Plant	Uḍumbara (*Ficus racemosa*)
Sacred diagram	Pañcacōnākāra Maṇḍala (pentagram)
Fasting	Friday
Mantra	AUM SHUKRAN SHUKRAYA NAMAHA – chanted 108 times at sunrise on Friday

Shani (Saturn)	
Alternate name/s	Saptārchī, Pangu, Manda or Sanaiścara
Associated deity	Yamaraj (lord of the underworld)
Gemstone	Blue sapphire (primary), blue amethyst (substitute)
Metal	Lead (Pb)
Colour	Blue
Grain	Tila dhanya (sesame seed)
Plant	Shami (*Prosopis cineraria*)
Sacred diagram	Dhanurākāra Maṇḍala (archway)
Fasting	Saturday
Mantra	AUM SHAN SHANAISCHARAYA NAMAHA – chanted 108 times at sunrise on Saturday

Rāhu (Northern Node)	
Alternate name/s	Abhra-pisācha, Kabandha or Hastā-bhū
Associated deity	Sarpa (serpent god)
Gemstone	Garnet/cinnamon stone
Metal	Brass (Cu+Zn)
Colour	Blue
Grain	Masha dhanya (black gram)
Plant	Dūrvā grass (*Cynodon dactylon*)
Sacred diagram	Sūrpa karnākāra Maṇḍala (winnowing basket)
Fasting	As Saturn
Mantra	AUM RAM RAHAVE NAMAHA – chanted 108 times at sunrise on Saturday

Ketu (Southern Node)	
Alternate name/s	Dānava, Munda, Akacha or Aslesha-bhava
Associated deity	Chitrāgupta (keeper of Akashic records)
Gemstone	Chrysoberyl/cat's eye
Metal	Bronze[45] (Cu+Sn)
Colour	Variegated
Grain	Kulatha (horsegram)
Plant	Kusha grass (*Desmostachya bipinnata*)
Sacred diagram	Dwajākāra Maṇḍala (flag)
Fasting	As Mars
Mantra	AUM KE KETAVE NAMAHA – chanted 108 times at sunrise on Tuesday

CONCLUSION

Recent decades have shown a surge of interest in many of the occult sciences; perhaps none more so than palmistry and astrology. This reawakening has stirred considerable curiosity in all forms of Vedic wisdom; not only Hastā Rekha, but in all of its sister-sciences such as Āyurveda, Yoga, Vāstu, Rasa Shāstra and more. In this book I've tried to give some account of the richness embedded in the science of Hastā Rekha Shāstra. I therefore am hopeful that the information contained in this book will inspire others to explore the hand and palm, searching out its symbols of destiny.

NOTES

1. Rasaratnasamuchaya (9th century AD) considers pañcamaharatna to be: ruby, emerald, topaz, sapphire and diamond.
2. Kauṭilya's *Arthashāstra* includes one of the earliest commentaries on Rantashāstra (gemmology).
3. *Garuda Purāṇa*, one of 18 major religious texts. There appears to be no agreement on the historical age of the Purāṇas though references have been made to them as early as 550 BCE. This Purāṇa states the following gemstones to be a prophylactic against snake/insect bites, and diseases: Padmaraga (pink ruby Al_2O_3), Tarkshya (emerald $Be_3Al_2SiO_6$), Indranila (blue sapphire Al_2O_3), Vaidurya (chrysoberyl $BeAl_2O_4$), Pushparaga (topaz Al_2SiO_4), Vajra (diamond C), Mukti (pearl $CaCO_3$), Karketana (possibly a type of quartz), Pulaka (realgar As_2S_2), Rudhirakhya (blood stone SiO_2), Sphatika/Bhisma stone (quartz SiO_2) and Pravala (red coral $CaCO_3$).
4. Authored by Varāhamihira, c.450–570 CE.
5. Varāhamihira likens varieties of diamond to: Indrā, Yama, Vishnu, Varuna and Vāyu, etc.
6. Describing itself as 'A Gospel Book of Hindu Astrology with Master Key to Divination', the date of BPHS remains problematic, but is estimated to be in the region of AD 300–600. Our modern BPHS appears to have been recompiled late into the 19th century and contain a number of anomalies, such as unequal house systems, remedial measures and Jaimini techniques.
7. BPHS Chapter 3 ('Planetary Characters and their Descriptions') makes reference to metal/gemstone and lunar nodes, stating that lead and blue 'gem' are to be assigned respectively.
8. Indian alchemical literature, known as *Rasa Shāstra*, reached its golden age on or around the tenth century AD. Rasa here refers to the use of the metal mercury (Hg) to transmute base metals into gold as well as to transmute the bodily tissues into gold (everlasting and untarnished). For more information, see the author's previous work: *Rasa Shāstra: The Hidden Art of Medical Alchemy* (Mason 2014).
9. *Caraka Saṃhitā* acknowledges some gemstones to have anti-visha (anti-poison) properties, that is, to protect the wearer against snake bite. Recommended maṇi include: ruby, pearl, emerald, diamond and lapis lazuli.
10. Literally, a compendium of mercury and gemstones by Vāgbhaṭāchārya, c.9th–13th century AD.
11. Only the highest quality gems are suitable for bhasma. Gemstones should be glossy, bright, highly rayed, clear, heavy, well formed and bright coloured. Dull, scratched, cracked, broken, contaminated (with other minerals or bubbles) gems are to be considered unfit for medicinal purposes.
12. Red Spinel ($MgAl_2O_4$) is found in Śrī Laṇkā and used as a substitute for red coral.
13. Hessonite/Garnet ($Ca_3Al_2(SiO_4)_3$, known also as Cinnamon Stone.
14. Rulership of Diamond relates to colour imperfections. Clear diamonds are given to Shukra (Venus), whereas copper coloured are given to the Sun, blue to Varuna, brown to Indrā, yellow to Agnī, white to the Lord of Pitris and green-coloured specimens to the Maruts. Those whose colouration is similar to conch are worn by Brahmā.
15. A mixture of milk, yoghurt, ghee, honey and jaggery.
16. Pearls are often graded on a four-tiered system: (A) = low grade, misshapen; (AA) = ovular, 20% or surface blemishes; (AA+) = oval, 90% blemish-free; (AAA) = spherical, high lustre, 95% blemish-free metallic surface. Pearls suitable for astrological purposes should be AA+ or AAA grade.
17. Carnelian (SiO_2 + Fe) or Spinel (also known as Balas Ruby) $MgAl_2O_4$ can be used.
18. Highest and most rarefied tissue in the body. There is no direct correlation in modern medicine but Ojas can be thought of as supporting the immune system and maintaining bodily strength and health.

19. Bala = strength.
20. Intense spiritual practices.
21. Also known as Śuddhaspaṭika.
22. A red sulphide of arsenic.
23. Sapta = seven and Dhātu = tissues.
24. Unaffected by intense heating or oxidisation. Iron also features in this group but probably for its resistance to high temperature, its strength and medicinal properties.
25. After repeated heating these metals start to oxidise.
26. Tainted or mixed.
27. In some instances Sun is considered warrior caste and the Moon merchant caste.
28. The lunar nodes are sometimes awarded servant caste, but are more commonly associated with the king's militia (recruited for war en masse).
29. A scraping, licking action.
30. Pottali means to bundle or wrap in a packet.
31. Also yanthra.
32. Suraya (also kavacha), protective talisman worn to empower/negate planetary rays.
33. Known in India as Yajnopaveeta.
34. Also sutra.
35. Other popular sutta include Karaniya Metta Sutta, Rathana Sutta and Maha Mangala Sutta.
36. *Callicarpa macrophylla*, used in Āyurveda to alleviate excess Pitta and Vāta, that is, diabetes, dysentery, fevers and tumour reduction. Priyangu is astringent, sweet and pungent in taste.
37. Anjana = stibnite (Sb_2S_3), antimony trisulphide.
38. *Butea monosperma*, a popular Āyurvedic herb, associated with the Moon. Known as the 'Flame of the Forest', this herb works well on relieving excess Pitta/Kapha dosha. Primarily a bitter herb, it cleanses the eyes, kidneys, liver and spleen. It also shows affinity to asthi-dhātu (bones and joints). Symbolically its association with Ketu Graha may be due to its appearance, reminiscent of the reddening lunar disc during a lunar eclipse by Ketu.
39. Yukthi = applying logic, Vyapa = alternate, Ashraya = source
40. Satwa = essence/purity and avajaya = to attain/overcome adversity
41. Mantra, sacrifice or devotional acts performed before a sacred fire.
42. Vedic ritual.
43. Ritual for alleviation of malefic planets including incense, exotic foods, herbs, spices, fire and, in some cases, animal sacrifices.
44. Fire (sacrificial) ritual.
45. Wearing of gemstones for astrological purposes.
46. Varta Loha (also Pañca Loha or Pasloha) is another metal attributed to Ketu; this alloy contains equal quantities of copper, bronze, brass, iron and lead.

Appendix

THE BAJAJ SEER (AN INTRODUCTION TO VEDIC PALMISTRY)

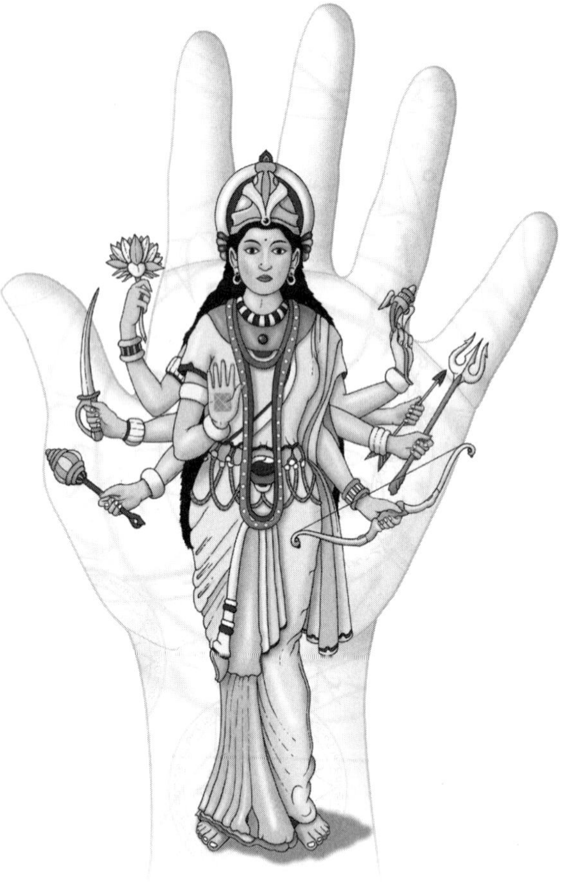

Pañcāṅgulī Devi (goddess of Vedic Palmistry).

ॐ वं रं हं सः पंचांगुली महादेवी श्री श्री मनोधर शासने अधिष्ठात्री
करन्यासौ शक्तीः श्री धृतीः श्रुतीः ॐ वं रं हं सः

Auṃ vaṃ raṃ haṃ saḥ Pañcāṅgulī mahādevī śrī śrī manodhara śāsane
adhiṣṭhātrī karanyāsau śaktīḥ śrī dhṛtīḥ śrutīḥ aum vaṃ raṃ haṃ saḥ

Translation:
Auṃ vaṃ raṃ haṃ saḥ – great goddess of five fingers and prosperity (Pañcāṅgulī), bestower of power and knowledge of sacred scripture, who in her teachings brings clarity to Rekha (lines upon the hand) and stability of mind – auṃ vaṃ raṃ haṃ saḥ.

Vedic Palmistry landed squarely in my lap in the spring of 2005, after embarking on an extended period of Āyurvedic study. As it happened, fate had already diverted me from an Indian destination to that of its close southerly neighbour, Śrī Laṇkā. Stepping off a plane on 24 December 2004, I checked in, unpacked and had barely re-orientated myself before a world-headlining Tsunami slammed into the island's south-eastern coastline.

Watching the populace get thrown into a national emergency and frenzied panic, I began to wonder if I'd made the right decision to be in this part of the world at this time. I resolved to push onward, trying to make the most of my internship in a small privately run Āyurvedic hospital, deep in Colombo 8, my new home until the end of the following year.

SETTLING IN 2005

Muted New Year's celebrations came and went while the island seemed to settle a little, life returning (I was told) to its normal manic pace. As the influx of volunteers, rescue workers and aid began to ebb, beach properties along the devastated south coast once again began to resemble tourist resorts. The last of the scattered debris was broken up, burned or buried.

My primary residence was a small room above the Āyurvedic clinic/dispensary. This facility was run by a collaboration of dedicated doctors, each specialists in their own field. The establishment offered patients a number of outpatient treatments including *Pañca Karma,*[1] *Shalakya Tantra* (minor surgery), *Vajikarana* (fertility clinic), a diabetes management clinic, a weight loss clinic and a beauty spa, as well as a number of western-trained GPs.

Weeks and then a month slipped by and although my schedule was somewhat flexible, I felt the need to keep a sense of urgency – not to succumb to the heat or the laid-back (almost horizontal) pace of life. The only break in the day's routine was to sit in front of my laptop for a few hours. Up until this point it had performed without incident, but suddenly decided to fail in spectacular style, dying at the most inopportune of moments. I found myself staring (open-mouthed) at the dreaded blue-screen-of-death, as it was in those days.

Watching a solitary cursor winking at me from the corner of the screen and daring me to press another key, the enormity of the situation slowly sank in. Of course, at home with laptop manuals, spare parts and an IT whizz at the end of a phone, this sort thing could be annoying – but in my current situation was a totally new order of frustration. Colombo 8 was one of the less affluent parts of the city and I was still feeling my way about. I had the additional advantage of not being able to speak a word of Sinhala, all of which made this particular situation seem borderline hopeless.

Shutting down the computer, I closed the lid and looked out of the window. What now, I thought, watching a few kids playing cricket in a nearby dust-bowl. No point moping in my room, I concluded, there was nothing for it but to have a drink at the local café – which luckily was a few short steps from my room.

At that time the clinic boasted a small café near its entrance and wandering downstairs looking like a kid who'd had their bike stolen, I ordered *Divul*,[2] slumped into one of the uncomfortable plastic garden chairs and chewed over my options. Divul smoothies were the best thing on the menu but alas were not on the house; none the less, they were worth every rupee. I sat taking a few cooling sips.

Suddenly, I became aware of another figure in the café, snoozing in a chair nearby with his forehead pressed against the tabletop. This, I realised, was the café's chef, obviously taking forty winks after the morning's graft. I half let out a chuckle, only to rouse the poor fellow, who raised his head half bewildered. Realising it was only the foreign student, he relaxed and intimated whether I required anything from the bar. I raised my drink, he smiled and resumed his stupor. As the clinic's only resident student, I was still a bit of a novelty. While most of the doctors spoke good English, the staff were slightly more difficult to communicate with – it was for the most part pretty hard work. If I kept sentences short and made lots of hand gestures I could get through the day without too much hassle. I guess on this occasion my dejected look and mannerism spoke volumes, and he figured even though I had my drink there was something amiss.

'Why?' he said, raising his hand in a twisting motion (a very typical Śrī Laṇkān thing to do).

'Laptop,' I said, accompanied by my downward pointing thumb.

'Shop,' he said, pointing toward the street.

'In the city,' I affirmed, nodding – yes.

'Nooo,' he said, still pointing across the street at the adjacent private residences, or what I had taken to be so.

On this point he seemed quite adamant and, as I followed his pointing finger, what I'd taken to be a private residence did in fact start to look a little more like a retail outlet. Through its darkened windows I began to see the silhouettes of electrical equipment and components. Like many of the high street shops in this district, lights were typically switched off until a customer wandered in, becoming almost emblazoned if you had cash to spend.

A well-faded banner above the entrance displayed a company name half hidden by late morning shadows. Closer examination revealed one of the words to be *Computer*! Things were finally looking up. Curiosity prompted me to hurriedly finish my drink before crossing the busy main road outside the clinic. Thanking our friendly chef for his tip, I darted back upstairs, scooped up my laptop and headed out into traffic, dust and a cacophony of car horns.

A CHANCE MEETING

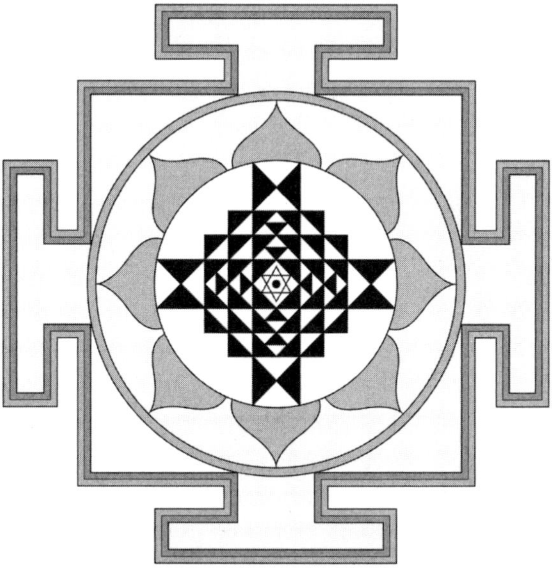

Pañcāṅgulī Yantra.

As I stepped across the store's dusty threshold, its interior revealed a veritable Aladdin's Cave, precariously stacked from floor to ceiling with computer accessories, cardboard boxes and advertising boards. The shop was really like a TARDIS: pokey from the outside, but considerably spacious once inside.

Almost immediately a young sales assistant greeted me, eying the laptop under my arm. His English was pretty good and his knowledge of computers excellent. I briefly explained my predicament while trying to coax the machine to life. After encountering the same scenario I let him try his luck, his nimble fingers trying a number of diagnostic procedures – all to no avail. After minutes of unsuccessful key tapping, he straightened and stood a while in thought.

'Not software problem, hardware – I think, it's quite new, yes? There's warranty?' he said. The laptop was still under its original international one-year warranty.

'We need to look inside' he said. 'Our engineer will diagnose, then advise.'

'How long will it take?' I asked.

'We look now,' he said.

And with that, he disappeared into a back room with my machine.

Killing time, I began wandering about the store, pulling items off shelves, poking various gadgets or tapping keyboards. At the rear of the shop I spied a second assistant perched at a half-hidden computer. From where I stood it looked like he was merrily surfing the internet. Now that my status had been escalated to 'prospective customer' I wondered if I'd be in a position to ask if I might check my email. I figured the worst he could do would be to say 'no', but to my surprise he got up and motioned me toward the screen. Very trusting, thought I – but also confirming my suspicion that he was in fact just taking a little time out of his day to surf. He'd evidently been following my movements and seen his co-worker engage me.

After scanning my mail I was about to vacate when my eye fell on a postcard amongst sticky Post-it notes plastered at the top left of the screen. The once-lavish technicolour print clearly showed a Hindu goddess, obviously connected to palmistry, her palm outstretched, revealing a horoscope inscribed thereon. The background of the image, though slightly menacing, revealed a hand with lines glowing like a futuristic circuit board. When the second assistant returned, I asked him where I might get a copy of the card. He told me the postcard (and computer) belonged to the company accountant, a man we'll identify as Mr. S. I commented how out of place the card was, in amongst all the hi-tech in-store toys. The assistant laughed and said Mr. S was a real character, excellent with money and obsessed with palmistry.

'Is he any good at foretelling the future?' I asked.

'He is accurate,' said the second assistant, 'but I do not believe in such things.'

At which point assistant number one returned with an irritated look on his face. Speaking a few short words in Sinhala to his co-worker, he turned to me.

'Definitely hardware problem – graphics card. We need a new card, it will take one week,' he said.

'Then go ahead. I could really use this thing fixed ASAP,' I said, and was about to give him my address when we were both drowned out by the sound of a Bajaj motorcycle[3] – with non-existent baffles.

Turning, I saw a rather large figure outside the shop dismount and stow his crash helmet. The rider then proceeded to enter the shop and plod slowly over to where we had congregated, sitting down at the computer I'd been using. Adjusting his spectacles, he tapped the keyboard without acknowledging any of us, pausing only to raise his hand in annoyance (presumably finding something amiss). Swivelling in his seat, he looked over the top of glasses and aimed a few choice words at the two assistants.

This, I surmised, must be Mr. S, 'company accountant', and now obviously complaining about unauthorised computer use in his absence. The tail-end of the complaint was in English – maybe for my benefit, he added, 'This computer is for accounts, not internet.' He complemented the last words with an upward spiralling hand gesture.

Ignoring the accountant's comments, the first assistant carried on where he'd left off and said, 'We need information' and with that disappeared in the direction he'd come, leaving us (the second assistant and me) with the sullen accountant. Looking a little sheepish, as I'd been the last one using his PC, I took the opportunity to lighten the mood, again enquiring about the postcard attached to the computer.

'I like your postcard,' I said nodding toward at the wrathful-looking deity, bearing a formidable array of weapons in her many arms.

Following my gaze, the accountant turned his head toward the card, then turned back to face me. 'They are fixing your computer?'

'Attempting to fix,' I said.

I then took the opportunity to explain my presence in the store and apologise for any disarray of his PC. I mentioned I'd borrowed his computer, checking emails and had noticed the postcard stuck to the screen.

'Is she connected to palmistry?' I asked.

'Are you interested in such things,' he said, beginning to mellow a little.

'I recognise some of the astrological motifs, and as palmistry and Jyotish seem to be inseparable in this part of the world I put two and two together,' I said.

'You have experience with Jyotish?' he asked.

'I was hoping to study a little here in Śrī Laṇkā, but so far I've not found time,' I said.

The accountant eyed his keyboard again and started to type, opening new documents. Just when it seemed our conversation was over, he appeared to have a change of heart and stopped typing. Looking up he said, 'Pancāṅgulī Devi, she promotes Hastā Rekha/palmistry.'

The first assistant, reappearing, handed me some paperwork. Jostling the papers I stared to focus on my original quest, asking for a pen with which to sign the necessary documents. The paperwork in my hand basically authorised the store to deal with the laptop's warranty. Mr. S passed me a pen from his pocket and I signed the papers where indicated.

Noting the discussion between myself and the accountant, the returning first assistant jokingly said, 'Did he tell you about your palm?'

'Nothing yet,' I said. 'How about you?'

'Oh, he is always telling and most often he is right. We are not asking anymore, he just says I told you!'

'They tell me your palmistry is very accurate,' I said to the accountant. 'Maybe I should ask you to look at my palm and tell me where I'm going wrong.'

'I am always telling here, but they do not or will not listen. Even when I am right, they make foolish mistakes, that is their nature. I have seen things on their hands,' said the accountant.

Turning in his chair, he took my arm at the wrist and, lifting his glasses, looked at my palm under the yellowing overhead strip-lights. Looking intently and muttering under his breath he then said, 'These matters are of a genuine interest to you.'

And then…he said, 'I did not want to teach at this time – but it seems I must.'

The accountant let go of my wrist and sat back in his chair with a rather serious look upon his face.

'I work four days each week. I start at 10 and leave at 6, I can give you 30 minutes at the end of each day. You must be punctual. Tomorrow I have an appointment, so we will start the day after?'

'I'm sorry, but are you offering to teach me palmistry?' I asked.

'Hastā Rekha Shāstra,' he corrected.

'But I thought you were analysing my palm,' I said.

'I did – and it seems I must teach you something of this,' he said.

The first assistant reached out and took the paperwork and started to walk back toward the main reception area. 'Do not worry about him,' he said. 'He is always that way.'

The remaining younger assistant gave an odd grimace as he began to restack items onto a nearby shelf.

'I'm happy to study, of course, but was not expecting the information in this manner,' I said. 'Luckily I'm staying right across the street, so...'

'Good,' said Mr. S abruptly, 'you will not be late.'

With that, he swivelled his chair to face the computer and resumed typing.

And so, just like that – all was arranged!

STUDYING PALMISTRY

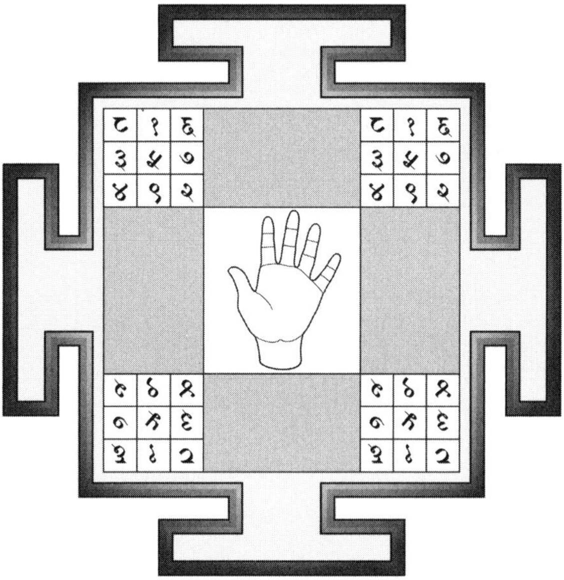

Hastā Rekha Yantra. Each of its four number boxes add up to 15, which then route to the number 6: (15) 1 + 5 = 6, or collectively (60) 15×4 = 60, 6 + 0 = 6.

As my studies progressed, I began to gain a richer insight into the hand and its various lines, understanding what they were able to reveal and what they could not reveal (as the case may be). My lessons lasted *exactly* thirty minutes; and four days in every seven, I crossed the street to receive instructions in the art of palmistry. At the close of each session I hurriedly returned to my room to collate my notes and try to reproduce the diagrams Mr. S had scribbled down during our time together.

During these lessons my tutor frequently took to drawing upon my palm with his pen, highlighting the lines that had powerfully influenced my life. This process was slightly annoying as I ended up with blackened palms; however, they did serve as a detailed record of our encounter and an excellent means with which to mind-map the palm in detail.

Amusingly (and a little scarily), Mr. S told me of people he knew who'd deliberately cut or burnt their palm, in an attempt to alter certain Rekha. This had been done mainly to thwart health issues or increase wealth attainment. Some, he said, drew daily upon the palm or cut lines, in an effort to bend the fates to their will. Others had done this as a daily reminder to stay focused on end goals.

'Does it work?' I jokingly asked.

'Sometimes – yes,' he said. 'Sometimes gain comes, but not always in a way they would choose. A man wanting wealth may instead have a terrible accident, but receive money for his injuries. It is bad practice to do these things, but it happens and works sometimes. Rekha show potential – like a map they indicate one way, but warn of problems along that way. So, in that way, better than map,' smiled Mr. S.

'If it's possible to modify fate by altering lines, I can see why people would be tempted to try, but you're saying that by doing so you run the risk of attracting more problems or perhaps depleting fortune promised in those areas,' I said.

'If Rekha become focused on, they burn up. Other Rekha will always try to balance. All Rekha show karma (action), but Karma Rekha (Fate Line) is best indication of fate. Interactions with this line or lack of interaction indicate likely events. Alternate hand must also be studied to assess *Purva-punya* (previous merit), as strong Rekha here promise long life, wealth, children, fame, etc.,' said Mr. S. (See Part I for a discussion on studying the alternate hand.)

REMEDIAL MEASURES

Broadly speaking, my studies were divided between the study of Rekha and Upaya (remedial measures). These, my tutor explained, were tried and tested means by which the palmist sought to placate (or enhance) the effects of planets.

Though some consider the use of remedial measures another form of wilful intervention, palmistry and astrology have a long tradition of applying techniques that have proven effective in the relief of *graha-apala* (malefic emanations of planets). The collective apparition of negative planetary forces is sometimes referred to as *sora*, *hora*, *saturu* and *bhaya*, that is, thieves, robbery, enemies and fear. Each inevitably seems to manifest the other, and islanders take their appearance (in any shape or form) to be perpetrated by unhappy planets. When dealt with in a timely manner, their potentially harmful cycle may be disbursed. Neglected or unappeased, planets are only noted to gain ground and intensity, eventually culminating in continual misfortunes.

Remedial measures feature prominently in Hastā Rekha, indicating their importance and acceptance in any understanding of this science. With a number of possible Upaya to choose from, it can be confusing to decide which option is best suited to the person before you. To make things a little simpler, I've highlighted five popular categories almost universally accepted as giving good results.

There are no hard and fast rules in the application of these techniques, as most appear to be based on personal experience or intuition. Personal circumstances surrounding the querent should also be taken into consideration, as some recommendations may be costly.

Note: Each of the following have been considered in greater detail in Chapter 12. For now I'll briefly identify the five categories as:

- *Gemstones/Maṇi:* Personal adornment of gemstones, or in some instances gems having been alchemically 'reduced' to a fine medicinal oxide (known as bhasma). Ingestion of these ashes allows the body to assimilate their properties without experiencing any toxic side-effects. Once assimilated, the residual effects of gemstones help ward off further instances of disease promoted by unruly planets.

- *Metals/Dhatu:* Akin to gemstones, planetary metals may also be worn to enhance or placate planets. Like gemstones, metals may also be alchemically transformed into relatively inert oxides. These may be taken internally as a bhasma. Metal wires are frequently interwoven to form bracelets or heated at higher temperature to form special alloys, which are then cast into amulets.

- *Talisman/Yantra:* Another popular method of planetary appeasement is construction of yantra and/or other protective talismans. These usually take the form of intricately inscribed copper sheets, rolled and worn in metal cases known as Suraya. To help reduce oxidation of the copper sheets, yantra are coated with specially prepared oils or the cases are sealed with mantra/prayers.

- *Sacred Sounds/Mantra:* Perhaps one of the most esoteric methods of planetary propitiation, mantra recitation is an ancient tradition whereby bīja[4] (sacred seed syllables) are repetitively chanted to relieve the effects of malefic planets. Mantra can be of varying length and complexity, and may also be multiple variations on similar themes.

- *Deity Worship/Deviyo-bandana:* Undertaken at a specific times of day ruled by a particular planet. Here, place, time and direction are set aside to propitiate one of the nine planets. Devotional acts such as prayer, meditation or self-sacrifice (that is, freely aiding or offering up time to advance a noble cause) are also considered an effective way to appease troublesome planets.

CONCLUSION

Classes ended abruptly one day as Mr. S announced that his office manager had decided to relocate him to another sector of the city. The locale change would henceforth make it impractical for him to maintain his teaching commitments. However, this sudden announcement was not to prove the end of the road for me, as I was able to locate alternative practitioners during my stay on the island.

During the interim, I came across a number of would-be teachers, but nothing of the calibre of Mr. S. I learned all too quickly the fatality of asking if anyone knew someone who knew a little palmistry – as that is exactly what you'd get, someone who knew 'little' about palmistry. One gentleman (with particular talent for bragging) insisted I study with him, as his knowledge was second to none. Foolishly, I took him at his word and paid up-front for a single lesson, only to sit and listen for one hour as he read to me from a book on western palmistry. I whiled away the hour looking at the end of my pencil and trying hard not to smile. The 'lesson' was not costly, but it did teach me another kind of lesson.

One methodology which proved quite rewarding was to speak with staff at the clinic, enquiring if they (or their immediate family) had had any positive experiences with local palmists/astrologers. Making a note of name and residence, I simply turned up and tried my luck. On the matter of teaching, most declined, or did not want to continually speak English; however, some did agree to teach – but in a limited capacity. Two such hopefuls were both skilled astrologers who happened to work with palmistry, both of whom insisted that their combination improved their hit rates. They also related to me the terribly vague nature of birth data amongst their clients, which was another good reason to rely more heavily on the palm. It was gratifying to have found these palmists/astrologers, and of course some of their techniques and ideas have partly contributed to the pages in this book. However, that being said, the more extensive knowledge of this science definitely belonged to Mr. S.

For my own part, I do not claim 'expert' status in Hastā Rekha and am grateful to have been given these opportunities to recognise *some* of the life-script written upon the hand. To date I have found Hastā Rekha Shāstra to be an invaluable adjunct to Jyotish, providing yet another vantage point from which to gaze upon past, present and future events. Little more can now be added to this tale, except to say that this book is an attempt to organise and reiterate the information imparted to me during my travels. I hope the reader finds the information to be of interest.

For those who feel a definite calling to the palm and its secrets, Pancāṅgulī Devi is most commonly propitiated during the lunar months of Phālgun and Chaitra, when Virgo Rashi and *Hastā Nakshatra* (see Chapter 10) dominate northern skies and host a waxing to full moon. Those wishing to gain mastery in Hastā Rekha are advised to recite her mantra seven times daily during these periods:

Auṃ vaṃ raṃ haṃ saḥ Pancāṅgulī mahādevī śrī śrī manodhara śāsane adhiṣṭhātrī karanyāsau śaktīḥ śrī dhṛtīḥ śrutīḥ aum vaṃ raṃ haṃ saḥ

Translation:
Auṃ vaṃ raṃ haṃ saḥ – great goddess of five fingers and prosperity (Pañcāṅgulī), bestower of power and knowledge of sacred scripture, who in her teachings brings clarity to Rekha (lines upon the hand) and stability of mind – auṃ vaṃ raṃ haṃ saḥ.

ENDNOTE

At the start of my first lesson with Mr. S, I asked him why he had taken it upon himself to instruct me, instead of just reading my palm (something he did eventually do and in which he was very accurate). He told me that my Rekha indicated to him the information disseminated would eventually propagate the wisdom of this science – perhaps a prediction that has to some extent been fulfilled?

NOTES

1. Pañca (five) karma (actions) is arguably the most powerful way to eliminate deep-seated toxins in the body.
2. A popular Śrī Laṇkān beverage made from wood apple (*Limonia acidissima*) mixed with jaggery, coconut milk and a little salt.
3. Bajaj Auto is one of the largest manufacturers of motorcycles, auto rickshaws and scooters in India.
4. There is no agreed meaning to seed syllables; their recitation is thought to provoke subtle (spiritual) energetics.

BIBLIOGRAPHY

Agrawal, B. (trans.) (2014) *Ravanā Saṃhitā (Mantra, Tantra and Yantra) Kali Kitib.* Based upon Uddish Mahatantra of Ravāna.

Birla, G.S. (2000) *Destiny in the Palm of Your Hand – Creating Your Future through Vedic Palmistry.* Merrimac, MA: Destiny.

Chidambaram Iyer, N. (trans.) (1884) *Brihat Samhita of Varaha Mihira.* Madura: South Indian Press. Available at https://ia601405.us.archive.org/24/items/bihatsahitvarah00iyergoog/bihatsahitvarah00iyergoog.pdf, accessed on 1 March 2017.

Chidambaram Iyer, N. (trans.) (1885) *Brihat Jataka of Varaha Mihira.* Madras: Foster Press. Available at https://ia902700.us.archive.org/1/items/brihatjatakavar00iyergoog/brihatjatakavar00iyergoog.pdf, accessed on 1 March 2017.

Dale, J.B. (1895) *Indian Palmistry.* London: Theosphical Publishing Society. Available at https://archive.org/details/indianpalmistry00daleiala, accessed on 1 March 2017.

DiCara, V. (with Kishor, V.) (2012) *27 Stars, 27 Gods – The Astrological Mythology of Ancient India.* London: Author, via Createspace Independent Publishing Platform.

Dwivedi, Dr. Bhojraj (2002) *Wonders of Palmistry.* Diamond Pocket Books.

Frawley, D. (1990) *The Astrology of the Seers: A Comprehensive Guide to Vedic Astrology.* Twin Lakes, WI: Lotus Press.

Frith, H., and Heron-Allen, E. (1886) *Palmistry or The Science of Reading: The Past, Present and Future.* London and New York: Routledge.

Gaffney, C.T. (1897) *Lessons in Palmistry, Studies of the Eye and Planetary Influences.* New York: Frederick A. Stokes. Available at https://archive.org/stream/lessonsinpalmist00gaff/lessonsinpalmist00gaff_djvu.txt, accessed on 1 March 2017.

Goravani, D. (2014) *Kārakas.* The Goravani Foundation.

Harness, D.M. (1999) *The Nakshatras, the Lunar Mansions of Vedic Astrology.* Twin Lakes, WI: Lotus Press.

Hathaway, E. (2012) *In Search of Destiny: Biography, History and Culture as Told through Vedic Astrology.* San Diego, CA: Vintage Vedic Press.

Kapoor, G.S. (2014) *Gems and Astrology: A Guide to Health, Happiness and Prosperity.* Rajan Publications.

Kapoor, G.S. (trans.) *Mantreswara's Phaladeepika.*

Kautilya (n.d.) *The Arthashastra.* London: Penguin Classics 2000.

Kirk, A. (2012) *Making Sense of Astrology.* Colombo, Sri Lanka: Lifelight 365.

Mason, A. (2014) *Rasa Shāstra: The Hidden Art of Medical Alchemy.* London: Singing Dragon.

Mason, A. (2017) *Jyotish: The Art of Vedic Astrology.* London: Singing Dragon.

Murthy, K.R.S. (trans.) (2003) *Vāgbhaṭa's Aṣṭāṅga Hṛdayam.*

Nārada Purāṇa (1950) Delhi, India.

Nath Dutt, M. (1908) *Garuda Purāṇam.* Calcutta: Society for the Resuscitation of Indian Literature. Available at https://archive.org/details/garudapuranam00duttgoog, accessed on 1 March 2017.

Roebuck, V.J. (1992) *The Circle of Stars.* Shaftesbury: Element.

Sharma, H.D. (ed.) (1933) *Samkhya Karika.* Available at www.universaltheosophy.com/sacred-texts/samkhya-karika, accessed on 1 March 2017.

Shubhakaran, K.T. (1991) *Nakshatra (Constellation) Based Predictions (With Remedial Measures).* New Delhi: Sagar.

Smith, V.A. (2009a) *Ayurvedic Medicine for Westerners. Vol. 1: Anatomy and Physiology in Ayurveda.* European Institute of Vedic Studies: www.atreya.com.
Smith, V.A. (2009b) *Ayurvedic Medicine for Westerners. Vol. 2: Pathology, Diagnosis and Treatment Approaches in Ayurveda.* European Institute of Vedic Studies: www.atreya.com.
Smith, V.A. (2009c) *Ayurvedic Medicine for Westerners. Vol. 3: Clinical Protocols and Treatments in Ayurveda.* European Institute of Vedic Studies: www.atreya.com.
Smith, V.A. (2009d) *Ayurvedic Medicine for Westerners. Vol. 4: Dravyaguna for Westerners.* European Institute of Vedic Studies: www.atreya.com.
Smith, V.A. (2009e) *Ayurvedic Medicine for Westerners. Vol. 5: Application of Ayurvedic Treatments.* European Institute of Vedic Studies: www.atreya.com.
Smith, I. (1901) *The Science of Palmistry and its Relations to Astrology and Phrenology.* Tacoma, WA: Author. Available at https://archive.org/details/scienceofpalmist00smit, accessed on 1 March 2017.
St. Hill, K. (1893) *The Grammar of Palmistry.* Philadelphia: Henry Altemus. Available at https://archive.org/details/grammarofpalmist00sthi, accessed on 1 March 2017.
Swami Krishna, T. (transliteration) (1901) *Shat Samudrika Shāstra.* Geneva Publishing Press, Chennai, Tamil Nadu.
Swami Modalari, K. (1909) *Nakshatra Chudamani.* Delhi: Gyan Books.
Toki, R. (2006) *Remedies in Astrology.*
Wilhelm, E. (2001) *Vault of the Heavens.* San Diego, CA: Kāla Occult Publishers.
Williams, L. (1902) *The Key to Palmistry.* Seattle, WA: International Institute of Science. Available at https://archive.org/stream/keytopalmistry00will/keytopalmistry00will_djvu.txt, accessed on 1 March 2017.
Wojtilla, G. (2009) 'Ratnashastra' in Kautilya's *Arthashastra. Acta Orientila Acadamiae* (Hungary).
Wujastyk, D. (2003) *The Roots of Ayurveda* (Revised edition). London: Penguin Classics.

RESOURCES

Palmist/hand reader

Johnny Fincham is a charismatic hand reader whose frequent media appearances and celebrity clients have made him widely known. Balancing modern techniques with intuition, his own particular brand of palmistry provides an excellent account of life experiences and of personality traits.
www.johnnyfincham.com

Āyurvedic study/consultations and Pooja services

Dr Venkata Narayana Joshi
Āyurvedic Consultations and Pooja Services
www.croydonayurvedacentre.co.uk

Dr Mauroof Athique (College of Āyurveda UK)
www.ayurvedacollege.co.uk

Vaidya Ātreya Smith (Āyurvedic Training)
Offering a three-level training programme to anyone interested in learning Āyurveda through advanced learning methods on an E-learning platform. Ātreya has been teaching since 1989 and his programmes are available for students all over the world.
www.atreya.com

INDEX